A
HOMEOPATHIC
HANDBOOK
OF
NATURAL
REMEDIES

A HOMEOPATHIC HANDBOOK OF NATURAL REMEDIES

—

SAFE AND EFFECTIVE TREATMENT OF COMMON AILMENTS AND INJURIES

—

LAURA JOSEPHSON, C.C.H., R.S.Hom. (NA)

VILLARD NEW YORK

The purpose of this book is to encourage the use of homeopathy
and other natural methods for the self-treatment of common ailments
and injuries. Before beginning to treat yourself or another, it is essential
to determine when a health condition is beyond your level of skill.
While knowledge gained from this book is designed to help you provide
ready and effective first-line care, it is not meant to be a substitute for
professional advice or medical treatment where these are appropriate
or required. If you are uncertain as to the seriousness of a condition,
or there is risk or danger to a person, always consult a health care
professional. Never treat serious injuries or ailments on your own,
or discontinue prescription medications without the advice of your
doctor. Homeopathy can still be an effective option after a visit
to your practitioner.

Published in the United States by Villard Books, an imprint of
The Random House Publishing Group, a division of Random
House, Inc., New York, and simultaneously in Canada by
Random House of Canada Limited, Toronto.

VILLARD and "V" CIRCLED Design are registered trademarks of
Random House, Inc.

Library of Congress Cataloging-in-Publication Data

Josephson, Laura.
A homeopathic handbook of natural remedies: safe and effective
treatment of common ailments and injuries / Laura Josephson.
    p.   cm.
Includes bibliographical references and index.
ISBN 978-0-8129-9188-8
1. Homeopathy.   2. Naturopathy.   I. Title.

RX76+   615.'32—dc21   2001051106

www.villard.com

Book design by Joseph Rutt

147028622

Dedicated to all the wise healers through the ages who have helped to illuminate for us the healing art and science of homeopathy; to today's homeopaths and those of the future who strive to carry the flame onward, lighting the way for generations to come.

And in remembrance of those who perished
on September 11, 2001:

Now that we've been shaken by death and destruction
Let us take the crude poison
And potentize it as a healing force
Let us breathe deeply the ashen air
And exhale it as sweet incense
So that love of neighbor and trust in God
May reign upon the earth

Laura Josephson
New York
October 9, 2001

ACKNOWLEDGMENTS

Many people have helped with the writing of this book. I would first like to thank my husband, David, and our four daughters for their immeasurable patience, love, and support, which enabled me to complete this project. To them I am deeply grateful.

I wish to thank Mary Bahr and Kathy Rosenbloom at Random House for their enthusiasm for this project. This book would not have been written without their interest and encouragement.

Special thanks are due to Sue Anello, C.C.H., and Jane Shepard, M.Ed., whose homeopathic knowledge, expertise, and friendship have been immensely helpful in gathering information and editing significant portions of the text.

My thanks also go to Estelle Delaunay and Danel Cove for their generous assistance and to many of my colleagues, dear friends, and family for their helpful feedback and kind wishes.

My gratitude goes as well to all the patients who have sought my help over the last ten years, whose trust and openness have been invaluable gifts. They have taught me much.

Last but not least, my heartfelt thanks go to the many devoted teachers in homeopathy and other fields, both living and departed, whose lives and work have inspired my own learning and love of homeopathy. Their dedication and courage to seek truth, wholeness, and healing continue to guide my daily steps.

CONTENTS

INTRODUCTION

The highest ideal of cure is the rapid, gentle, and permanent restoration of health; the removal and annihilation of the whole disease by the shortest, most reliable, and least harmful way, according to clearly comprehensible principles.
—Samuel Hahnemann, *Organon*,
6th edition

For as long as mankind has inhabited the earth, human beings have suffered afflictions and have sought healing. Remedies for our ills have been found by looking toward the natural world around us. The earth and its minerals, its waters, many plants, insects, and animals, and even the starry heavens have given humankind a rich array of tools through which we have learned diverse healing arts. Throughout evolution and up to the present day, we continue to blaze a trail through time, seeking to penetrate these very tools with human understanding, wisdom, and compassion.

Today that trail leads us on many divergent paths, some intersecting, some never to meet. Among these different roads, the widest and most traveled in the United States is the current conventional medical system. Much like an overcrowded airport terminal, this system is often congested, ineffectual, and overpriced; travelers often experience side effects, feel anonymous, and arrive at their destinations bewildered and exhausted.

On the journey to good health, more people today are in search of alternative routes that better meet their needs. In fact, these routes are rapidly widening as Americans beat a path to alternative and complementary medicine in increasing numbers. Today nearly *half* of all Americans use at least one alternative form of therapy.

Many people are looking for a healing method that respects and honors the inherent wisdom of the body and the individuality of each person, that stimulates the body's natural ability to heal itself, that utilizes powerful yet gentle natural remedies which produce no toxic side effects; in short, a healing system that understands true health to be an integrated wholeness of all human qualities.

Homeopathy is one such wise and gentle approach. For more than two hundred years homeopathy has helped people all over the world find solutions to their health problems. It is among the most accepted forms of natural medicine in the world today. According to the World Health Organization, homeopathy is the *second* most widely used system of medicine in the world and the fastest growing. It is well established in the United Kingdom, France, Germany, Russia, India, and many other countries around the world. For over a century the British royal family has preferred homeopathy to other forms of treatment, and the Queen of England retains a homeopathic physician. From minor ailments to more serious chronic diseases, homeopathy offers a sound science of healing based on a holistic view of the human being, that is, a system of care that takes the whole individual into account and does not just treat isolated symptoms.

It may be surprising to learn of the popularity that homeopathy enjoyed in the nineteenth and early twentieth centuries in the United States. Homeopathy's success in Europe spread to the States in the 1830s, and by the turn of the century approximately one in five of all physicians were homeopaths. At that time more than one hundred homeopathic training colleges and twenty medical schools flourished in the United States; more than one thousand pharmacies made and supplied homeopathic medicines. Homeopathy gained wide acceptance in part through its tremendous success in treating epidemic diseases, such as yellow fever, scarlet fever, and cholera.

At the same time, however, the American Medical Association (AMA) was trying to purge the profession of any physicians who practiced outside the conventional model. In fact, the AMA was founded in 1846 expressly in opposition to the increasingly popular homeopaths. In 1855 the AMA added a stipulation to its code of ethics that any doctor who consulted with a homeopathic physician could be expelled. The AMA persisted in its aim to suppress homeopathy. It influenced state licensing boards and medical college funding committees and collaborated with the financial interests of pharmaceutical companies to disparage homeopathy. The success of these efforts was substantial: After 1910 many homeopathic medical colleges lost funding and closed down or were converted into conventional medical schools. By 1950 no homeopathic medical colleges remained in the United States, and only an estimated one hundred practitioners were left. Despite the dismal decline, homeopathy remained alive through independent homeopathic study groups, a handful of dedicated practitioners and their patients, and connections to homeopathic circles in Europe and other parts of the world.

Over the last twenty years, with a widespread recognition of the flaws and limitations of conventional medicine, and with increased public interest in natural approaches, homeopathy has undergone a worldwide renaissance as people rediscover its benefits. Because of this homeopathic remedies are inexpensive and easy to obtain; homeopathic books, articles, studies, and other resources are widely available through booksellers and the Internet; and a variety of homeopathic schools and training programs are increasingly accessible to both health care professionals and the public.

The holistic approach found in homeopathy is especially relevant today. Mainstream twentieth-century medical thinking promoted a mechanistic model of the human being, in which health and illness are seen as primarily determined by the functioning of molecules, atoms, and biochemical interactions. The idea that nonphysical aspects of our makeup, such as human consciousness, are connected to physical health is an ancient concept but is relatively new in contemporary Western culture. Only in recent years has there been a heightened awareness of and interest in the mind-body connection. Many current studies provide evidence that physical health can be measurably transformed by practices such as meditation, prayer, artistic activity, and positive thinking. An integrated view of mind, emotions, and the body is a central aspect of healing with homeopathy and has been from its very beginnings.

Although a mechanized method of health care continues to dominate, many physicians and scientists today are coming to recognize the validity of a holistic view. The current system of overly specialized care puts us at risk of losing sight of the big picture. When, for example, a person takes one medication for high blood pressure, one for allergies, one for indigestion, and another for anxiety, he or she may get some temporary relief of symptoms, but this is by no means a cure. In this picture we see a model of health care that fails to take the person's overall well-being into account and falls short of truly restoring health. Excessive use of medicines may also cause further ailments in the form of unwanted side effects.

Whether prescribed singly or in combination, conventional drugs carry a far greater risk than do homeopathic medicines, whose risk is virtually nonexistent. According to a report published in the *Journal of the American Medical Association* in 1998, adverse reactions to correctly prescribed conventional drugs represent the *fifth* leading cause of death in the United States, accounting for approximately 140,000 deaths annually. Nearly one-third of these deaths are the results of drug interactions.

While conventional drugs and interventions do have their place and are appropriate in many situations (especially in emergencies and life-threatening conditions), it makes good sense to turn first to therapies that boost the immune system for the majority of common health problems. Recognizing and exercising our self-healing abilities by using homeopathy strengthens our immune systems. When used wisely and consistently, homeopathy will help to guard against the tendency to chronic diseases so common today. Ideally, homeopathy, other natural therapies, and conventional medicine should be used to complement one another in a way that best serves the unique needs of the individual.

While no single method of health care can meet everyone's needs all the time, homeopathy is an excellent first course of action not only in the treatment of short-term (acute) ailments but also for deeper, persistent (chronic) conditions. Homeopathy has a long history and a fine record of successfully treating chronic diseases. Not only for physical illnesses, homeopathy is capable of addressing a wide spectrum of mental and emotional problems as well: depression, anxiety, and learning and behavioral problems to name just a few.

Should you choose homeopathy for a chronic illness, do not attempt to treat yourself. Do seek the care of an expert homeopath, who is best equipped to manage such cases. Professional homeopathic treatment that addresses chronic or recurrent conditions as well as general preventive care is referred to as *constitutional treatment*. This type of care is suitable for a broad range of physical, mental, and emotional problems.

GOALS OF THIS BOOK

The goals of this book are to introduce to you the healing art of homeopathy and to enable you to use homeopathic remedies and other natural methods to treat common ailments and injuries. I sincerely hope that you will find this handbook a reliable, easy reference for use in a wide variety of health conditions. There are many situations in which you can safely and effectively use homeopathy with benefit while avoiding prescription and over-the-counter drugs.

The guidance given in this book is not intended to replace medical advice but rather to support you in giving natural, homeopathic care in relatively low-risk situations. Even in urgent conditions that require medical care, homeopathic remedies can be safely given en route to the emergency room or doctor's office.

This book can assist you in gaining a more confident, active role in taking care of yourself and your family. I always encourage individuals and families to cultivate a sense of responsibility for their own health while joining in a trusting partnership toward healing with the practitioners of their choice. I hope that your confidence to treat yourself and loved ones, as well as the partnership you have with your family physician or practitioner, will be enhanced by your reading of this book.

As you put into practice the guidelines set forth here, I hope you will be inspired and strengthened by the experience of knowing the body's ability to heal itself naturally. Homeopathy helps us to cure ourselves. Through homeopathy we have the potential to know ourselves better, to listen to and trust the wisdom of our remarkable human design.

Over the long term, when people become healthier through using homeopathy, they become ill less often, recover more quickly when they do get sick, and are less prone to chronic disease. As a result, the use of homeopathy will allow future generations to be healthier. Eventually, as homeopathy becomes more prevalent, we may reasonably hope to see a decrease in the incidence of chronic disease. Ultimately, my hope is that your own and your family's health will benefit in the broadest sense, and that this health benefit will be passed on to future generations.

May this handbook be a steady road map for your healing journey!

HOW TO USE THIS BOOK

Part 1 provides an explanation of the history and guiding principles of homeopathy, giving background and historical context for the modern home prescriber. Homeopathic terminology used throughout the book is explained both in Part 1 and in the glossary.

Part 2 provides guidelines for taking the case of an injured or ill person, from gathering information through reviewing the findings, selecting the right homeopathic remedy, choosing the potency, and administering the remedy. By following these guidelines you may find the most appropriate homeopathic treatment. The last portion of Part 2 contains a description of homeopathic remedies, tinctures, and ointments necessary for a well-stocked home kit.

The following three parts represent groups of ailments with their corresponding homeopathic treatments. Commonsense home care guidelines are also given where appropriate, as well as advice on when to seek professional care. Part 3 covers first-aid conditions; Part 4, acute ailments such as coughs, colds, flu, and stomach upset; and Part 5, common childhood conditions.

Part 6 contains the materia medica, or descriptions of the major homeopathic remedies recommended in the previous sections. Referring to this section will provide a fuller understanding of each remedy and help clarify your remedy selection.

This materia medica provides a reference to all the homeopathic remedies mentioned in this book with their common names. It is followed by a glossary of homeopathic terminology, a suggested readings list, a bibliography, and an Internet resources directory.

PART I

WHAT IS HOMEOPATHY AND HOW DOES IT WORK?

HISTORY AND
GUIDING PRINCIPLES

*A man could not be born alive and healthy were there not
already a physician in him.*
> —Paracelsus

*The softest things in the world overcome the hardest things in
the world.*
> —Lao-tzu

How remarkable it is that when we have a cut or wound on the skin,
our inner healing forces immediately rally to defend against infection,
create a protective scab, and heal the tissues beneath it. We have
all experienced this simple fact, yet it is amazing that our bodies accomplish this without any conscious effort on our part. Every human
being is endowed with inherent self-healing resources capable of
meeting a wide spectrum of physical, emotional, and mental stresses.
Homeopathy recognizes this inner physician working ceaselessly to
maintain health and balance in body, soul, and mind.

Homeopathy is a safe and effective system of medicine that helps
to restore health by stimulating the body's inherent ability to heal itself. This process is activated by giving medicines made from substances found in the animal, vegetable, and mineral kingdoms. Each
medicine, or remedy, is selected for its similarity to a sick person's

unique symptoms of illness or suffering. The word *homeopathy* is from the Greek: for "similar" (*homoios*) and "suffering" (*pathos*).

A wide range of conditions can be successfully treated with homeopathy: acute illnesses and infections, injuries, chronic diseases, and mental or emotional disorders. Whether in minor illness or in deeper disease, homeopathy recognizes that all symptoms of ill health are expressions of a disharmony within the whole person, and that *it is the person who needs treatment, not the disease*. Symptoms are seen not as the illness itself but as healthy signs that our defenses are managing an inner imbalance in the best possible manner under the circumstances. When given appropriately a homeopathic remedy has the power to gently restore health and vitality on all levels: physically, emotionally, and mentally.

HAHNEMANN AND THE LAW OF SIMILARS

In the late 1700s a German physician named Samuel Hahnemann (1755–1843) developed the medical science and art known as *homeopathy*. Like Hippocrates two thousand years earlier, Hahnemann recognized two methods of treating illness: one by way of opposites and the other, preferred method, by way of similars. The conventional medical system of today, called *allopathy* or *allopathic medicine*, treats by way of opposites.

The fundamental law upon which homeopathy is based is the *law of similars*, which states: Let likes be cured with likes, in Latin: *Similia similibus curentur*. This means that a remedy can cure a disease if it produces in a healthy person symptoms similar to those of the sick person. Therefore, homeopathic treatment involves giving a sick person a substance that would cause the very same symptoms of illness in a healthy person.

For example, we all know that slicing onions can result in burning, watery eyes and a runny nose; but when red onion is given as the homeopathic remedy known as *Allium cepa*, it is curative for people who suffer from hay fever or common colds and share those particular symptoms. Likewise, we know that drinking too much coffee can cause a person to feel restless, nervous, overstimulated, and unable to sleep; but a homeopathic dose of *Coffea cruda* is curative for people with insomnia and other nervous conditions that share these characteristics. Hahnemann would nod in agreement with the spirit of the adage, "Take a hair of the dog that bit you."

Hahnemann was the first in modern times to test the law of similars and create from it a scientific method of treating illness. However, he did not claim to have discovered this concept. The law of similars has roots that can be traced to the cultures of ancient India, China, and Greece. In 400 B.C., Hippocrates described this natural law: "Through the like, disease is produced, and through the application of the like, disease is cured." Paracelsus, the sixteenth-century German physician whose writings would later influence Hahnemann, described this principle as well.

Hahnemann did not come by this knowledge without considerable personal and professional trials. He had been a highly respected physician and author of texts on chemistry when, despite his accomplishments, he felt increasingly disturbed by the brutal medical practices of his time. Bloodletting, purging, and toxic doses of mercury and arsenic were popular treatments. His conscience would not allow him to remain silent, and he became an outspoken critic of the system that he thought did more harm than good. His colleagues were quick to denounce him as a medical heretic, and as his frustration grew he eventually withdrew from the practice of medicine. To support his growing family he turned to translating medical treatises. However, he remained faithful to his hope of discovering "if God had not indeed given some law . . . whereby the diseases of mankind would be cured."

While working on the translation of a medical text by William Cullen, a renowned Scottish professor of medicine, Hahnemann stumbled upon an assertion that was to become the key to fulfilling his hope. Cullen claimed that cinchona bark, or quinine, was an effective cure for malaria because of its bitter and astringent qualities. Hahnemann was astonished and doubtful of this because he knew of many equally bitter substances that did not cure malaria. But he felt compelled to investigate Cullen's assertion and, in the true spirit of scientific inquiry, decided to test the effects of cinchona bark on himself. After taking successive small doses of the substance, he developed a reaction: his array of symptoms was strikingly similar to those of malaria. Hahnemann deduced that the curative power of cinchona bark lay not in its bitter qualities but in its ability to create the symptoms of malaria in a healthy person. This experiment was the first homeopathic proving.

PROVINGS

Hahnemann continued to research other substances in the same manner. A circle of friends, followers, and colleagues grew around him, and with their assistance he went on to establish a comprehensive program of testing potentially curative substances on healthy volunteers. This process is called a *proving*. Amid the gathering momentum he also found himself once again practicing medicine, now applying the law of similars to treating the sick.

In the provings of Hahnemann's time as well as those of today, a group of healthy people is given extremely small doses of a single substance over a period of days until symptoms unlike their normal states develop. Each person carefully records in detail symptoms he or she experiences. All the provers' symptoms are then gathered together to form a *remedy picture*. This list represents the most consistently experienced range of symptoms from among the provers, "as if one person." By this method the medicinal effect of a substance can be determined for therapeutic use.

Information from provings is then gathered with data from toxicological reports and accidental poisonings when applicable. The combined data is entered into a reference book called a *materia medica*

(Latin for "materials of medicine"). Referred to by all homeopaths, the materia medica lists all the homeopathic remedies in use. It describes in detail the mental, emotional, and physical symptoms associated with each medicinal substance.

At the time of Hahnemann's death in 1843, he had completed provings of ninety-nine substances and written six editions of the *Organon*, his guidebook for the use of homeopathic remedies. By the end of the nineteenth century, over six hundred more remedies were added to the list of proven medicines. Today there are over thirteen hundred remedies registered in the *Homeopathic Pharmacopoea of the United States*.

THE MINIMUM DOSE

Hahnemann firmly believed in the importance of using only the minimum amount of a medicine to effect a cure. He called this the *principle of the minimum dose*. Since human beings are by nature endowed with strong healing forces, Hahnemann thought that only a small stimulus should be necessary to begin the process of cure.

Giving the smallest dose of a remedy acts as a catalyst to a person's own defenses. Once the healing action has begun, the process is allowed to continue on its own to "overcome and destroy the existing disease without further ado," as Hahnemann put it. That is, without giving any more medicine than is necessary. The same remedy may be repeated on an "as needed" basis depending on the vitality of the person, the nature of the illness, and the individual's overall response to each previous dose. The guiding principle is: Always give the least amount of medicine required for healing. A person may expect to end the course of medication upon feeling well, without having to "finish the bottle." In this we see the ideal of restoring health without a perpetual dependency on taking medicine.

THE SINGLE REMEDY

The use of one single remedy at a time is another basic principle and is the hallmark of what is called *classical homeopathy*. Contrary to the common convention of taking two or more medicines at a time, a person does not need to take one homeopathic remedy for headache, a different one for gas, and yet another for anxiety because, as mentioned earlier, it is the person and not the disease that is to be cured. Though a person may have any number of mental, emotional, and physical symptoms, that person has only *one* disease: his or her own singular susceptibility and disharmony. Therefore there will be only one remedy picture that will most closely match the overall *symptom picture* of the person.

TOTALITY OF SYMPTOMS

As stated earlier, a single remedy is selected to match closely a person's whole symptom picture, called the *totality of symptoms*. It is essential to take this totality into account in order to select the most effective remedy. This totality includes not only the obvious symptoms of the chief complaint but a variety of other characteristics as well. Even symptoms that may seem small or unrelated to the main complaint can be crucial to the ultimate choice of remedy, because they can point to a person's underlying susceptibility or other critical factors.

Indeed the word *symptom* can be defined as any perceptible change in the mental, emotional, and physical well-being of a person. For example, changes in appetite and thirst, sensitivity to heat and cold, energy level, sleep and dreams, peculiar sensations, temperament, and mood all may contribute to the totality of symptoms. Part 2 includes a more extensive explanation of symptoms. Thus, the totality is the broadest possible view of the ill person's symptoms.

POTENTIZATION: HOW REMEDIES ARE PREPARED

Hahnemann's patients began responding quite well to the new form of treatment. However, he was concerned about the toxic side effects some patients experienced. He hoped that giving even smaller doses might remove the side effects. He began to experiment with diluting medicines in increments until the side effects were removed. At first he was disappointed when the medicines appeared to lose their effectiveness. Then he discovered that by vigorously shaking the solution and diluting it alternately in progressive steps, he was able to attain results that exceeded his expectations. Not only were the side effects gone but his patients were restored to health more quickly than before.

Hahnemann called this method of preparing medicines *potentization*. He was able to produce many new medicines in this manner, from a variety of mineral, plant, and animal sources. Still used today, this process allows some of the most poisonous substances known in nature, such as arsenic and snake venoms, to be rendered not only harmless but into health-restoring medicines, in a sense turning swords into plowshares.

By adding the step of shaking the solution, which Hahnemann called *succussion*, the dynamic force of the medicine was increased, and through dilution the risk of toxicity was eliminated. Much to his amazement, the more highly diluted and succussed substances acted more powerfully in curing his patients. Some of the most brilliant results came from potencies so high that no perceptible amount of the original substance was left. How was this possible?

How potentized remedies work is still difficult to explain in concrete scientific terms. We are so accustomed to the idea that more is better—in drug terms, the more milligrams the better the cure. But there is clearly an energetic principle at work in healing with homeopathy, one reason why it has aptly been called energy medicine. Homeopaths recognize that remedies act by what may be called the vibrational imprint or energetic impression of the original substance. Although the material evidence in potentized remedies may not be readily visible under a microscope, their results form a clearly recognizable phenomenon for anyone who has seen or experienced healing with homeopathy.

Numerous examples from physics and biology confirm the power of infinitesimally small substances, such as trace elements. Within the human body these essential substances are barely detectable, yet their absence would result in serious illness. We also know that thyroid hormone is present in our blood at only one part per 10 billion yet is sufficient to regulate our entire metabolism.

Research conducted recently at the California Institute of Technology points to the validity of potentization. The study tracked changes in water molecules as they underwent the dilution and shaking process when single substances were introduced. The usually random water molecules began to form distinct clusters that exactly mimicked the shape and form of the original substance. The more diluted the solution, the bigger and stronger these clusters were, leaving a lasting "imprint" in the water—despite the fact that no original substance remained. (See "Homeopathy: Dilute and Heal," by Andy Patrizio, *www.wired.com*.)

We must also consider that scientists have difficulty explaining numerous phenomena that are accepted as perfectly serviceable, for example, aspirin or the immune system. No one has actually seen an immune system, only its effects. In a materialistic society some skeptics dismiss homeopathy because of potentization, on the grounds that what you can't see isn't there, and that the remedies must work only by a placebo effect. The placebo effect, however, would not account for the well-documented success of homeopathy in treating epidemic diseases, such as numerous cholera outbreaks in the United States and abroad. Nor would the power of suggestion account for how effective homeopathic remedies are in treating babies and animals, who would presumably not be suggestible. Although potentization may appear veiled in mystery, the results of well-prescribed homeopathic remedies are not. Homeopathic remedies may be infinitesimally small, but their effects are sizable. It is *the quality, not the quantity* of medicine that truly makes the healing difference.

Today all homeopathic remedies are standardized and prepared by homeopathic pharmacies according to the strict guidelines set by Hahnemann. The remedies are available in a variety of strengths, or potencies.

The most common potencies for home use range from lower to higher: 6, 12, 30, and 200. The higher the number, the stronger the potency, and the further the remedy has been diluted and succussed. The number is followed by either a C, for example, 12C; or an X, as in 12X. The C and X represent different scales of dilution; that is, how many parts of water were mixed with the original substance. One scale is centesimal (one to one hundred); the other is decimal (one to ten). Remedies of 200C potency are used mainly by professionals and are seldom recommended for the home prescriber. Professionals may use even higher potencies, millesimal (dilution factor of one thousand), such as 1M, 10M, 50M, and CM. These are considered high or very high and are administered only by expert homeopaths in severe acute conditions or during constitutional treatment.

Remedies are prepared by homeopathic pharmacies in the forms of tablets, pellets, globules, or pills of varying size, depending on the manufacturer. They are most commonly available in a lactose (milk sugar) or sucrose base and are instilled with the remedy solution. Liquid remedies preserved in alcohol are also available from some homeopathic pharmacies. Further information about potencies and administering remedies can be found in Part 2.

A HOMEOPATHIC VIEW
OF HEALTH AND DISEASE

We live in the lap of immense intelligence, which makes us
receivers of its truth and organs of its activity.
                        —Ralph Waldo Emerson

THE VITAL FORCE

As stated earlier, all human beings have inherent self-healing capaci-
ties. This is because of the existence of what Hahnemann called the
vital force, the ever-present, nonmaterial life energy that is a part of
each human being, and indeed every living thing. Referred to in
other traditions as the life force, life body, or etheric body, which is in
Oriental medicine akin to *chi* or *qi*, the vital force is the dynamic
principle that perpetually maintains the form and function of each
living thing: "that energy which distinguishes living things from non-
living things," as Hahnemann described. Without the vital force the
physical body has no animation, no feeling, no life. The vital force
also operates as the "memory body" of our past illnesses and injuries,
as well as past and present habits.

Our defense mechanism or immune system is the self-protecting
aspect of the vital force, which allows us to be self-regulating and au-
tomatically compensates for disruptions or changes in our environment. For example, we cough after inhaling dust, we perspire when
overheated, we produce a scab when we have a cut or a wound. Symptoms, therefore, arise as a result of the vital force's best efforts to

defend against stresses. Illness manifests when the vital force is susceptible to certain stresses.

When a homeopathic remedy is given, it acts directly on the vital force, as one energetic phenomenon interacting with another. The similarity or resonance between the state of the human vital force and the remedy's vibration is *the* factor that stimulates the healing process. Our vital force or life energy determines whether we are healthy or ill. It thus makes sense that energy medicine would help restore us. Balanced diet, adequate rest, exercise, and a healthy mental and emotional outlook are among other crucial factors that support the vital force and ultimately the healing process.

WHAT IS HEALTH?

Health is more than the absence of a diagnosable illness. Many people today who might describe themselves as being well would also say that they aren't exactly healthy either. From a homeopathic viewpoint, health is defined in much broader terms than it would be by average standards. Simply speaking, optimal health means the ability to withstand a wide variety of stressors.

According to the homeopathic view, health encompasses three interrelated elements of our human makeup: the physical body, the emotional or feeling life, and the thinking or mental sphere. When we are in excellent health, these elements coexist in a harmonious way that allows us to be adaptable and flexible within a wide range of conditions. When a person is healthy, there is an inner sense of balance, freedom, and creativity; a sense of contentment or well-being physically, emotionally, and mentally. His or her vitality becomes like a well-tuned instrument through which the music or spirit of the person may shine forth. Whether stress comes from the outer environment or is generated within, an optimally healthy person is capable of rebounding from life's challenges with relative ease and speed. Any limitation or impairment of the three aspects may be considered an obstacle to overall health.

WHAT IS ILLNESS?

Illness occurs as the result of a weakness or imbalance in the body's defenses. This imbalance produces physical, emotional, and mental changes that are different from a person's normal or healthy state. These changes we call symptoms. One may say that the imbalance *is* itself the illness, and the eventual manifestation of symptoms is the *result* of that prior imbalance. In homeopathy there is an understanding that this inner disharmony precedes the appearance of illness.

Many types of stress can cause illness, but whether an individual becomes ill depends on his or her susceptibility. Exposure to inclement weather, environmental toxins, overexertion, loss of sleep, poor diet, mental strain, grief, and disappointment are a few examples of factors that can lead to illness. Hereditary factors also play a role. Each person has his or her own unique predispositions or susceptibilities.

For example, during an outbreak of the flu, many people can be equally exposed to the virus, but only some will actually become ill. Some will have mild symptoms, while others may develop more severe symptoms. Why? Susceptibility is the factor that determines whether someone falls ill and with what intensity.

The meaning of illness has occupied human thought for thousands of years. A full exploration of this question is beyond the scope of this book. However, the meaning of illness plays an influential role in determining what we hope for in a cure.

It is worth considering briefly that *it is the nature of illness that our inner resources be challenged to struggle in some way.* Toward what end? At intervals throughout the unfolding drama of life, we are brought face-to-face with inner aspects of our being that are blocked or stuck. Like a river obstructed by a boulder, our life's course may be able to bend around an obstacle until it becomes too clogged with debris. The water swells behind the blockage, pressure builds, and there is stagnation. When nothing flows illness develops. Bailing out some water may reduce the swelling, but only temporarily. Clearing away the surrounding debris may also give relief, until it builds up again. To truly restore the dynamic flow, however, the obstacle must be removed. Only then may the river carry on its course, its destiny.

Illness may be seen as an opportunity to struggle with and eventually dislodge that obstacle, moving us toward a better state of health in body, soul, and mind. So illness may be viewed as a gift or a blessing, as an opportunity for transformation. We dishonor that gift by denying it with suppressive treatments, temporarily removing symptoms without addressing the underlying cause. We affirm the body's wisdom by motivating our inherent healing forces to cleanse, reorder, and put aright what is out of balance. Homeopathy allows us the possibility of transformative healing.

Illness can also be seen as a kind of practical schooling or education for the immune system. Childhood illnesses, for instance, are necessary milestones that play a vital role in providing immune benefits to last the course of life. Most childhood illnesses can be managed effectively with homeopathy and other commonsense natural methods, thus stimulating immune enhancement. It does not serve a child well to routinely suppress inflammatory illnesses with antibiotics and fever-reducing drugs. A discussion of these effects and the role that vaccines play in the health of the immune system can be found in Part 5.

WHAT IS A CURE? HERING'S LAW

Curing is much more than removing symptoms. Taking a conventional painkiller for headache or menstrual cramps will suppress or remove particular symptoms for a time but does not effect a cure. *Cure* is the full restoration of health, from the inside out.

A German homeopathic physician named Constantine Hering (1800–1880) gained much insight into the process of cure through his many years of clinical observation. He was able to ascertain three guiding characteristics of the healing process, which today is called Hering's *law of cure*. Hering was a renowned teacher of homeopaths and a great pioneer of provings. He settled in Philadelphia in the early 1830s, founded the Hahnemann Medical College there, and is considered the father of American homeopathy.

Today we can use Hering's formula as a simple way of observing and evaluating whether the process of cure is heading in the right direction. Hering's law is applied primarily in the treatment of chronic illnesses but is also useful for assessing the healing process in acute ailments and even in injuries, such as broken bones.

CURING OCCURS FROM THE INSIDE TO THE OUTSIDE. During the process of cure, the person will begin to feel a general improvement inwardly, with the innermost parts of the body being cured first. First there is increased energy and well-being, and finally the outermost aspects or peripheral symptoms of the physical illness are cured. Occasionally, shortly after the administration of the remedy, the person may feel like sleeping. After a nap or a night of sound sleep, there is improvement. Even though symptoms of illness may still be present, a boost in energy or the person's own sense of vitality is a good sign that the healing process is in motion. With a cold, for instance, the person is likely to feel better and consider the expulsion of mucus a welcome cleansing rather than a nuisance.

CURING OCCURS FROM ABOVE TO BELOW. Symptoms disappear starting from the upper part of the body and proceeding downward. In the case of a rash, for example, eruptions would first disappear from the head and face, and clearing would gradually move down the body, passing last through the hands and feet.

CURING OCCURS IN THE REVERSE ORDER IN WHICH SYMPTOMS APPEARED. Symptoms of a previous illness may resurface during the healing process. This often happens in the reverse order of the original sequence. For example, a child with asthma may have at one time been treated with cortisone for eczema. During homeopathic treatment, as the asthma improves the eczema may reappear after having been suppressed. The skin symptoms will eventually be removed during the healing process.

This last aspect of Hering's law is most often observed in the treatment of chronic illness but can be relevant to acute cases as well. If a related symptom from a past injury or illness reappears during acute treatment, this may be an opportunity to clear out the dormant remains of that imbalance. As long as there is overall improvement, the older symptoms may clear up on their own. It is best to wait until all forward progress halts before considering another dose of the current or a new remedy.

SUPPRESSION OF SYMPTOMS VERSUS CURE

The homeopathic ideal of cure is that a person should ultimately become strengthened by the experience of his or her own vital force overcoming the illness. *A person should be more well after an illness is resolved than before the illness appeared.* This does not happen, for example, in the case of a child whose fevers are routinely suppressed with aspirin or acetaminophen (Tylenol), when antibiotics are given with every earache or antacids are used habitually for indigestion. Conventional medicines often suppress symptoms so that the illness appears to recede, but they do not stimulate the vital force, much to the person's detriment. *Suppression is the missed opportunity for the expression of illness to find its vent.* An imbalance cannot find its way out of the human organism and is pushed deeper inside. There it will hide, eventually to show itself again, or worse, it becomes a deeper form of illness. Such is the consequence of suppression: The immune system does not "learn" through experience that it can overcome illness and is weakened gradually by suppression, inviting the possibility of even more illness. One could say that our suffering is in vain if we do not make use of our own healing forces during illness.

The idea that the suppression of symptoms is unhealthy is quite foreign to the conventional medical view. Most of us have been raised with the notion that as long as a symptom (such as pain, fever, rash, discharge) can be suppressed, we are healthy. But this approach has far-reaching negative consequences. The evolution of disease through human history is marked by suppressive treatments that have led to deeper states of illness. Sweeping the dust under the rug does not make for a clean house. The ideal of cure is to remove the underlying cause, that is, to lift the rug and clear away what is unwanted.

PART 2

PUTTING HOMEOPATHY INTO PRACTICE

TAKING THE CASE

The world is full of obvious things which nobody . . . ever observes.

> —Sherlock Holmes, in *The Hound of the Baskervilles*, by Sir Arthur Conan Doyle

The universe is made of stories, not atoms.

> —Muriel Rukeyser, American poet

Everyone has a story to tell. In illness and in health each of us carries a remarkably diverse collection of attributes that make up the unique story of who we are. To use homeopathy effectively, perceiving and understanding a sick person's story is of the greatest importance.

Unlike conventional medicine, homeopathy does not rely on laboratory tests to assess most illnesses, and even the definitive "diagnosis" or particular name for a condition is of limited use. Instead, there is a trust in the wisdom that the human constitution will communicate what is needed for healing through the symptoms it produces. The person as an individual, not the disease, is what we should most closely observe. The production of symptoms is a healthy sign that the person's defenses are managing an inner imbalance in the best possible manner under the present circumstances.

Illness is expressed in a unique way by each person. For example, five people with sore throats may each require a different remedy.

One person's sore throat may develop quickly along with a fever and a flushed face. Another may have aching pain on one side only, which develops slowly without fever. Yet another will have a particular stinging pain with swelling in the throat. Careful observation of those individualizing symptoms will lead the prescriber to an understanding of the sick person's unique story and ultimately to the correct remedy. Once a case is well understood, what remains is to match the totality of the symptoms with the most similar homeopathic substance. Then an appropriate remedy may be selected and given.

Case taking is the process of gathering information through listening, questioning, and careful observation. Reviewing the findings is second, and finally comes selecting the remedy.

Whether you are taking the case of another adult, a child, or yourself, it is best to write everything down, as much as possible in the sick person's own words. Keep a health file or notebook with a section for each family member or friend you treat. Recording dates, symptoms, remedies given, and results can make future treatment much easier, especially if a particular condition should recur.

In taking the case of someone who is ill, you will need to use all your senses to gather information, as a good detective would. You will see, hear, touch, and even smell out the case. Aside from physical symptoms, illness is often accompanied by mental and emotional changes. Anything that tells you about changes in the ill person can be considered a symptom, but the more unique to the person the symptom is, the more importance it has.

For example, we all know that in the common cold typical symptoms include a stuffy or runny nose, sneezing, perhaps sinus pain or headache. To find the correct remedy, however, it is most helpful also to know the distinctive way the sick person has changed from his healthy condition to the way he expresses his common cold symptoms. Is the nasal congestion relieved in the fresh air or does it become worse outside? Is he more thirsty or thirstless? Does he want cold or hot drinks? Is he dry or perspiring? What color and consistency is the nasal discharge? Is he restless, more irritable and touchy, or mild and prone to tears? Is there a particular time of day when he feels much worse? These and other distinctive features will help to draw the fullest and clearest picture.

Before and during case taking, observe the person's mannerisms and emotional demeanor. First impressions may reveal many clues. Once you've begun, allow the person to describe the condition in his or her own words without interrupting. It is best to question only as necessary, avoiding the use of suggestive or leading phrases. For example, ask, "What kinds of drinks soothe your throat?" or "Do you prefer your drinks hot, cold, room temperature, or with ice?" instead of "Do hot drinks soothe your throat?" Simply gather the information through careful listening, questioning, and observation. If you think of a particular remedy while you are taking notes, avoid coming to a conclusion too soon. Jot down your idea and save it for when you review the case.

If you are the one who is ill, case taking can be more challenging, depending on the ailment and how you are feeling. When assessing your own condition, try to rely most heavily on indisputable symptoms, such as strong physical ones. In this way, if your judgment is clouded by your illness, you can still make a reliable remedy choice. Emotional nuances and mental states are often the most difficult aspects of oneself to be objective about. If you are finding this assessment especially challenging, ask for clues from family or friends who may see you more objectively.

Someone who is ill or injured may struggle with responding to questions or describing an ailment. For instance, during fever, confusion or delirium may prevent the person from describing her symptoms clearly. This in itself may be one of the symptoms upon which you eventually prescribe.

The basic tenet taught in journalism schools rings true with case taking: Always find out the who, what, when, where, why, and how. Here is a summary of information you will need to gather to form a well-taken case:

CAUSATIVE FACTORS: Did the illness begin after a particular situation? Examples: exposure to weather conditions, such as being in a cold, dry wind or becoming wet; overindulgence in food, alcohol, or drugs; loss of sleep; emotional stresses, such as receiving bad news, grief, embarrassment, anger, or fright; mental stresses, such as overwork or overstudy. Sometimes a person has "never been well since" a particular injury, illness, or event. You may need to dig around a bit to find the original stress, but do not belabor the point; pinpointing a causative factor may not be possible. In this instance just proceed with taking the case.

ONSET AND CHRONOLOGY OF ILLNESS OR CONDITION: How long has the condition been present? Did symptoms develop slowly or rapidly? Have they changed much since the onset? Sometimes a person will skip around chronologically while telling his or her symptoms. Make sure you understand the evolution of the condition in the right order.

LOCATION: Where exactly is the pain or discomfort? If there is any ambiguity, keep asking until you are absolutely sure. Have the person point to the area to clarify if necessary. Do pains radiate or extend from one place to another? Is one side of the body affected more than the other? For example, with a fever, is one cheek red and the other pale?

CHARACTERISTICS: What does the pain or discomfort feel like? Ask the person to describe the sensations as fully as possible, for example, dull, aching, burning, stinging, sharp, squeezing, cramping, heavy, bursting, numb, or tingling. Also consider "as if" symptoms, such as "it feels like a load of bricks on my chest," "dizziness as if the whole room is spinning," or "it's like there's sand in my eye."

MODALITIES: Any influence or factor that either improves or worsens any of the symptoms is called a *modality*. What circumstances make the condition better or worse? For example, being in fresh air or a closed room, before or during a thunderstorm, in the sun, time of day or night, sitting, lying in a particular position, motion or rest, after sleep, periodically (for instance, between 4:00 and 8:00 P.M., every spring, once a week), before or after eating, while swallowing or talking, when alone or in company. Does the person feel better or worse from being touched? In the case of backache or headache, does she desire firm or light pressure, or is she averse to touch?

GENERAL SYMPTOMS: Aside from the localized symptoms, how has the illness affected the person in a general way? Is he warmer or chillier than usual? Are there changes in appetite or thirst, new food cravings or aversions? Are there changes in sleep, or in mental or emotional states? How is the person's overall level of energy or fatigue?

THE ART AND SCIENCE OF OBSERVATION

Our observations and sense impressions are essential in taking a case, and what our senses tell us varies from person to person. What we perceive and how we interpret it depend largely on the combination of our subjective and objective orientation. This is one reason homeopathy is both a science and an art. Hahnemann advised that one strive to be objective in case taking, to be "an unprejudiced observer," to seek the truth, free from bias. In addition to the five senses, we may utilize what we commonly call our *intuitive sense*, which can be an invaluable tool when used judiciously and supported by our objective findings.

Here is an illustration of how each sense is used to gather information for the case.

SIGHT: Observe facial expression and color; posture, gait, and movement. Have a look at the tongue: Is it clean or coated white or yellow, streaked, cracked, or patchy? Is the person's general appearance tidy or messy? Also take note of the sick person's surroundings when applicable. Is the window open or a fan on, or is he heaped with blankets in a warm, closed room? Is he alert and sitting up, or slumped down in the chair or bed?

HEARING: Are there changes in voice, manner of speech, and breathing or sighing? Is a cough deep, wet, barking, dry? Does the person moan or talk in her sleep? When a child cries, is the sound piercing and sharp, sad and pitiful, or angry sounding? Is the person very talkative, or does the silence tell you that she is averse to speaking? Listen with care to her choice of words and emphasis on particular aspects of her condition. She may offer descriptive analogies such as "I've got a lump in my throat" or "It feels like a knife in my back when I bend down." Such descriptions can be invaluable clues. Further, you can observe if the person has trouble finding the right words or has difficulty speaking.

TOUCH: Touch the skin to feel if it is dry or sweaty, cool or warm. During fever is one part of the body hot while another is cool? Compare your sense of touch with what the person describes; for example, does he say that he feels very hot though his skin is cool to the touch? How does the person react to being touched?

SMELL: On entering the sick person's room, is there a strong odor? Is it sour, musty, offensive, garlicky, or sweet? Are there changes in the odor of the breath, body, stool, or urine? If you are not sure, ask the person or caretaker whether he or she has noticed such changes.

OVERALL SENSE OF THE PERSON: What do you sense that has changed about the person's mental or emotional state? Do you notice mental dullness, excitement, forgetfulness, confusion, disorientation, or delirium? Do you detect marked emotional states, such as anxiety, fearfulness, irritability, anger, sadness, despair, or indifference? These are but a handful of mental and emotional symptoms that may be part of the whole symptom picture. When you are gathering these symptoms, your intuition can come into play. Using your intuition is fine, as long as you stay focused on allowing only what is true about the person to enter the case. Often there will be one or more physical symptoms to support intuitive findings.

In some instances finding the simple truth about a person can be challenging. Have patience with yourself as you develop your case-taking skills. If you find that your emotional reactions to a patient make it difficult for you to be unbiased, ask someone close to the person to confirm your perceptions. The effort to engage all the senses in the service of truth will aid you in understanding a person more fully and objectively, and increase the likelihood of successful treatment.

REVIEWING THE FINDINGS AND SELECTING THE REMEDY

Now that you have so diligently taken the case, it is time to interpret your findings. In reviewing the case you will need to identify which symptoms are significant. Evaluate them as you look over your notes, applying the following questions:

- What is the intensity of particular symptoms? Which symptoms "speak the loudest"?

- With what force or strength have the symptoms changed from the person's healthy state?

- Which symptoms most strongly limit the person's ability to function in a normal way?

- Which symptoms are unusual or peculiar to this type of ailment, or to the specific person?

Go through your notes and circle the symptoms that stand out most substantially. It is best to select at least three symptoms that strongly and clearly represent the case. In homeopathy we use the metaphor of having a three-legged stool on which to rest the case. The three legs of the stool are indisputable physical, emotional, or mental symptoms. It is ideal to choose a symptom from each of these legs; however, *any* combination of indisputable symptoms can make a good case as long as the totality of symptoms is well represented.

Next, look up the condition under the appropriate heading and review the remedy options listed. Select the one remedy that is most similar to the overall picture of the illness.

If you need more information to differentiate between remedies, turn to the materia medica in Part 6 for fuller descriptions of the more prominent remedies. These will help you distinguish more accurately the features of each remedy. For instance, when differentiating between cough remedies, if the affected person is extremely irritable and ill-tempered, you could discount *Pulsatilla* as a possible remedy because, as you will read, people who need *Pulsatilla* are generally sweet and mild-tempered. It is important to remember that *all* the symptoms listed for a remedy do *not* have to be present for the prescription to be correct. Indeed it is extremely rare that a person's illness contains all the symptoms described. It is necessary, though, that the remedy be very similar to the picture of the illness. You may wish to supplement the information in this book with a more extensive materia medica, which contains a larger number of remedy descriptions in greater detail. (See the suggested readings at the end of this book.)

If you are still unclear about which remedy to select, or if you can find no strongly indicated remedy, do not give a remedy. It is always best to avoid giving any type of medicine when its use is not truly indicated. In this case, give other natural supportive measures when applicable and consult a professional homeopath or other health care provider. It is a wise caregiver who knows when and where to turn for help. Some may feel this is a failure on their part, but in fact it is praiseworthy to know one's limitations, especially when the health of others is concerned.

Here are two sample cases that illustrate the selection of the remedy, as well as potency and repetition of the dose, to be discussed in the following section.

SAMPLE CASE 1

A child plays outside for hours on a chilly day. Shortly after he comes indoors at four o'clock, his face becomes flushed; he suddenly develops a high fever and becomes very anxious, restless, and fearful. *Aconite* is the most similar remedy that matches the child's suffering. *Aconite* 12C is given every fifteen to thirty minutes for three doses. His symptoms improve with each dose but relapse quickly, so 30C is given every twenty to thirty minutes for two more doses. The fever, as well as the anxiety, restlessness, and fear, begin to abate steadily. Another dose is given an hour later, and a final dose is given two hours after that. By nine o'clock the fever is gone and he is able to sleep peacefully. His parents know that if he wakes during the night with any relapsing symptoms, another dose of *Aconite* 30C will give him rest. He wakes in the morning feeling completely well.

SAMPLE CASE 2

A woman has been a bit weary and out of sorts for several days since receiving a piece of bad news. Her limbs feel heavy and leaden, and increasingly she aches all over, feels chilly, trembly, and generally fluish. Her spirits are depressed, and she wants to be left alone to lie quietly. Chills are running up and down her back, her eyes are droopy and aching, and her tongue feels thick and heavy, making her speech a bit slurred. The totality of symptoms forms a picture of *Gelsemium*. She takes *Gelsemium* 12C every two or three hours. After three doses she feels markedly better, but four hours later there is a slight return of her symptoms. She takes one more dose, feels completely well in body and spirits, and her symptoms do not return.

SELECTING THE
POTENCY AND DOSAGE

Once you have selected the remedy, the next step is to select the potency and frequency of the dose. Rigid dosage formulas are not given with homeopathic remedies as they are with allopathic drugs, such as the mandatory ten-day course of antibiotics so often prescribed for various infections. In homeopathy we are guided by the intensity of a person's illness and his or her individual response to the remedy when determining the potency and repetition of the dose.

If you are new to homeopathy, the best potencies to choose from are the lower to moderate strengths, 6C, 12C, and 30C. Among these 30C is the highest potency, and more accuracy is required when using it to obtain best results. If you are less experienced, I recommend using mainly 12C and some 6C; reserve 30C potencies for when you are more confident of your remedy choice. If you purchase a remedy kit, start with a 12C or 30C kit; you may add other potencies as needed.

As mentioned earlier, there are two scales of potencies: The C potencies (centesimal: as in 6C, 12C, and 30C) and the X potencies (decimal: such as 6X, 12X, and 30X), the latter being lower in strength. The X potencies are perfectly serviceable for milder conditions or when C potencies are unavailable. Here are their equivalent values:

$$6X = 3C$$
$$12X = 6C$$
$$24X = 12C$$

Follow these fundamental rules when selecting the potency and dose:

- Administer the *minimum dose* necessary to stimulate a healing response.

- Stop giving the remedy *when there is improvement;* if symptoms recur, repeat the remedy as needed.

- Decrease the frequency of doses as symptoms improve; the interval between doses lengthens as the person feels better.

- If the symptom picture changes, select a different remedy.

- If there is no improvement after a reasonable effort, discontinue the remedy and reevaluate the case. Select another remedy or seek professional advice.

Consider these factors when selecting the potency:

- The more forceful or rapid the onset of symptoms, the higher the potency needed and/or the more frequently the dose will need to be repeated.

- The higher the potency, the more deeply the remedy will act but the more accuracy is required to obtain favorable results.

- The less certainty you have about the remedy you've selected, the lower potency you should use, but the lower the potency, the more frequently the dose needs to be repeated.

How often will you need to repeat the dose? That depends on the urgency of the condition. Follow these dosage guidelines:

SERIOUS CONDITIONS: Injuries or illnesses that require urgent attention and are likely to be accompanied by marked pain or distress, for example, serious burns, head injuries, traumatic shock, serious insect bites, painful bladder or ear inflammations

Give one dose every five to thirty minutes, in the highest potency you are confident using or have available: 6C, 12C, or 30C. Repeat as needed according to the severity, more often with a lower potency.

MODERATELY SERIOUS CONDITIONS: Moderately distressing or less painful symptoms that are serious but not urgent yet definitely need same-day attention, for example, recurrent vomiting, troubling cough, rising fever, blistering poison ivy rash

Give one dose every one to two hours: 6C or 12C, more or less often according to the potency of the remedy and the severity of symptoms. A 30C potency may be given slightly less often, such as every three or four hours, if you feel certain about the remedy choice or if lower potencies are not on hand. Be guided by recurrence of symptoms.

LESS SERIOUS CONDITIONS: Symptoms accompanied by moderate discomfort that could wait between twenty-four and forty-eight hours to be treated, for example, sniffles, sore throat, sprains, teething discomfort, and milder forms of stomach upset, diarrhea, or constipation

Give one dose every four to eight hours: 6C or 12C, more or less often according to the potency of the remedy and the severity of symptoms. A 30C potency may be given slightly less often if you feel more certain about the remedy choice or if lower potencies are not on hand. Be guided by recurrence of symptoms.

MILD CONDITIONS: Symptoms less distressing and lingering (but not related to a chronic illness); focused primarily in the musculoskeletal system, for example, minor discomforts from overexertion or muscle strains, mild teething symptoms, or the later, recuperative stages of healing broken bones

Give one dose three or four times per day: 6X, 12X, or 6C for
up to seven days, longer if specified for a particular ailment.
Discontinue the remedy when there is marked improvement.

Homeopaths agree that choosing the right remedy is of greater importance than selecting a particular potency. If the remedy you need
is available only in a different potency than would be ideal, go ahead
and use it. The repetition of the dose may be adjusted accordingly.
The frequency, that is, how often a dose is repeated, is what makes the
difference. So, in the case of an acutely painful strained back, for instance, for which you would have preferred to give *Rhus toxicodendron*
30C every three or four hours but only 12C was available, you may
give *Rhus toxicodendron* 12C, every two or three hours. Contrary to
what one would expect with allopathic medicines, doubling the number of pellets will not increase the strength of the dose at all.

Remember: Give only one remedy at a time. *Stop giving the remedy*
when there is clear improvement, and repeat it as needed, usually at less
frequent intervals as improvement continues.

ASSESSING THE RESPONSE

To assess whether a remedy is working well, you should observe changes not only in the physical symptoms of illness but also in the person's overall level of energy and sense of well-being. As stated in the section on Hering's law of cure, sometimes the first signs of improvement come in the form of a change in energy or vitality, before symptoms such as coughing or a runny nose improve. If the person feels better inwardly, that is a good sign, and physical improvements are likely to follow. In this case the remedy should not be changed.

After the first dose has been given, you may begin to see an improvement. At times you may need to give several doses to see a healing response. Usually if there is no change for the better by the third or fourth dose, you should consider giving another remedy. If you feel certain that the remedy is correct and there has been slight improvement, you may give up to six doses. First, though, eliminate the possibility of any antidoting factors. (See the following chapter.)

Generally if there is no improvement after four doses, you should assume that the remedy is incorrect. There is no harm done, other than the fact that you have lost time and the illness may have worsened. Review your notes and see if another remedy better suits the person. If there had been an improvement but symptoms relapsed, repeat the same remedy as needed. Sometimes the remedy picture has changed from when you first took the case. In this instance another remedy is warranted. Retake the case and prescribe accordingly. If despite your best efforts symptoms persist, worsen, or keep relapsing, seek professional advice.

HOMEOPATHIC AGGRAVATIONS

Occasionally symptoms may worsen slightly at the beginning of the healing process. The main complaint may intensify for a short time or a related symptom from an old illness may resurface temporarily as the body works to clear the illness from the inside out. This is a *healing crisis* or, in homeopathic terms, a *homeopathic aggravation*. With such an aggravation there is often a temporary increase in discharges. Physically there might be greater production of phlegm, perspiration, urine, or loose stools. Emotionally there may be tears. In whatever form is appropriate to the illness, discharges are the body's way of detoxifying, or "cleaning house." The ill person almost always feels better inwardly during an aggravation, often welcoming the cleansing effect of the outward symptoms. As the aggravation passes in most cases there is rapid and steady improvement. If the person experiences new symptoms after taking a remedy, the wrong remedy has been selected.

It should be stressed that aggravations do not occur in all cases, and they are more typically seen in the treatment of chronic illnesses when high potencies (200C, 1M, or higher) are used. For this reason it is best to use moderate to low potencies (30C or lower) for self-guided treatment.

WHAT TO AVOID

Some influences are known to interfere with the action of homeopathic remedies and can cause what is known as *antidoting*. Many homeopaths differ about which factors present the greatest risks of antidoting, but most agree that the following influences have interfered with treatment in a significant number of people. The occurence of antidoting depends in part on a person's sensitivity or susceptibility. So whether a remedy has been administered or is still in its container, and to ensure the effectiveness of homeopathic remedies, it is best to avoid exposing either the person being treated or the remedy to the following:

CAMPHOR OR MINT: These are ingredients in many salves and cosmetics, including Tiger Balm, Vicks VapoRub, Ben-Gay, Noxzema, Blistex, Carmex, and Sea Breeze. Personal care products that contain significant amounts of menthol, wintergreen, and eucalyptus—strong mint toothpastes, mouthwashes, and lozenges—should be avoided. All these substances are known to have an antidoting effect. Tea tree oil may also inactivate remedies.

STRONG ODORS: Strong odors either in the mouth or in the environment at the time of taking a remedy can affect its action. Therefore a remedy should be taken with a clean mouth, free from strong odors or flavors. Intense environmental odors, such as chlorine bleach, ammonia, mothballs, and paint solvents, may interfere as well. Subtle aromas from these agents are not usually a risk except among highly sensitive individuals.

EXTREMES OF HEAT AND COLD, AND DIRECT SUNLIGHT: Freezing temperatures or extreme heat may adversely affect remedies, so don't leave remedies in your car for extended periods during temperature extremes. Direct sunlight has been known to diminish remedies' effectiveness, so don't keep them on a sunny windowsill. Indirect daylight does not pose a problem.

COFFEE: Consuming coffee in large amounts, and in some cases moderate amounts, can have an antidotal effect. Drink decaffeinated coffee if you must. Better yet, drink tea (caffeinated tea is fine) moderately during homeopathic treatment.

STREET DRUGS OR RECREATIONAL DRUGS: Drugs including marijuana and excessive amounts of alcohol may also adversely affect a remedy.

MAJOR DENTAL WORK, X RAYS, AND MRIs: Ultrasonic dental cleaning and high-speed drilling have been especially known to block the effects of homeopathic remedies. Some people find that major X rays, CAT scans, and MRIs can interfere as well. If any such procedures become necessary while you are taking a remedy, you may need to increase the frequency of the dose or repeat it after the work is completed. Observe your mental, emotional, and physical state to see if there has been a change.

ELECTRIC BLANKETS: The electromagnetic field that surrounds a person while using an electric blanket is never healthful. The body's regenerative processes are especially active during sleep and are disturbed by such an influence. If you must use an electric blanket, prewarm the bed and unplug the cord before going to sleep.

OTHER HOLISTIC TREATMENTS: Though many other holistic therapies are perfectly valid unto themselves, combining certain treatments with homeopathy can be problematic. Acupuncture, polarity therapy, aromatherapy, and the use of magnets are best avoided while taking a homeopathic remedy. In some cases acupuncture may be used concurrently with homeopathy, but this combination is discouraged because of the difficulty in ascertaining which treatment is effecting changes. Unless your acupuncturist is well versed in both modalities, their combined use is not recommended.

If antidoting influences cannot be helped during treatment, be guided by common sense to ascertain whether a remedy's action has been diminished. Did the person experience improvement while taking the remedy and then begin feeling much worse after such an exposure? If so, give the remedy again, and repeat as needed if the response is good. If antidoting factors remain, a temporary lifestyle change may be necessary if homeopathy is to be effective.

ADMINISTERING THE REMEDY

Homeopathic pellets come in a variety of sizes, from poppy seed–size granules through moderately sized globules to larger tablets. No matter which pellet size you are using, the basic rule of thumb is that one dose equals a *pea-size portion*. So if you have the larger tablets, take one; with the medium-size globules, take two; if you have tiny granules, take the amount that will cover the bottom of the vial cap. A small, pea-size portion is all that is necessary for one dose, even if on the remedy bottle it says to take more. Even if you took the whole vial at once, the strength of the dose would not be increased at all. One dose is one dose, no matter the size. Bear in mind that what counts is the *quality* and the *frequency* of the dose, not the *quantity* of pellets. Homeopathic remedies work best when taken with a clean mouth. A remedy should be given at least fifteen minutes before or after eating, drinking, smoking, chewing gum, or brushing the teeth (drinking water is fine). This is meant as a general guideline; of course, in urgent situations do not wait for the minutes to tick by. In an emergency by all means give the remedy at once!

The remedy is administered by putting the pellets under the tongue. Tap the appropriate number of pellets into the vial cap, drop the remedy into the mouth, and allow it to dissolve slowly without chewing or swallowing. To ensure the remedy's effectiveness, follow these precautions:

- Avoid handling the remedy directly with the fingers, especially if you are giving the dose to another person. Sometimes with children and animals it is difficult to avoid handling the remedies. Do the best you can.

- If you've dispensed extra pellets into the cap, carefully tap them back into the vial.

- If any pellets accidentally fall, discard them.

- Always replace the vial cap promptly and securely.

- Never open more than one vial at a time.

- Be sure you have read about antidoting factors in the section titled "What to Avoid."

For people averse to lactose pellets, sucrose pellets or liquid remedies in alcohol are available.

BEING PREPARED: STOCKING AND STORING YOUR HOME KIT

The home medicine chest is a very personal thing. Each household traditionally has its collection of internal and external treatments to suit individual needs. I encourage you to think about the kinds of ailments you want to treat, sort out what you already have in your medicine chest, and put things in good order.

You will need to keep your basic first aid supplies well stocked. Items such as tweezers and scissors, rubbing alcohol, hydrogen peroxide, bandages, gauze, surgical tape, sterile cotton balls, compress cloths, ice pack, and hot water bottle are all necessities. Keep an illustrated first aid manual with your kit.

The following assortment of internal remedies, as well as tinctures, ointments, oils, and gels, will help you be prepared for a wide range of conditions. Also listed are some kitchen supplies that can often be useful.

The first group of internal remedies is essential for first aid, including more urgent ailments (such as food poisoning). The second group is for typically less urgent conditions, ones that can wait long enough for you to obtain a remedy as needed. These you should add to your kit at your convenience.

If you can afford it, purchase all the remedies at one time. A number of homeopathic sources sell premade kits containing from twelve to fifty remedies. Often these are less expensive in the long run than buying remedies one at a time. I recommend a 12C or 30C kit, to which you may add some selected 30C and 6C potencies. *Aconite* 30C and *Belladonna* 30C should be included and are especially valuable in the treatment of children. *Arnica montana* 30C and 200C should be added as well.

HOMEOPATHIC REMEDIES FOR YOUR HOME KIT

INTERNAL REMEDY GROUP 1: FIRST AID AND URGENT CONDITIONS

Keep on hand

Aconite
Apis mellifica
Arnica montana
Arsenicum album
Belladonna
Carbo vegetabilis
Cantharis
Hypericum
Ledum palustre
Rhus toxicodendron

INTERNAL REMEDY GROUP 2: LESS URGENT CONDITIONS

May be added as needed

Bryonia alba
Chamomilla
Dulcamara
Eupatorium perfoliatum
Ferrum phosphoricum

Gelsemium

Hepar sulphuris calcareum

Ignatia amara

Ipecacuanha

Magnesia phosphorica

Mercurius vivus

Nux vomica

Phosphorus

Pulsatilla

Ruta graveolens

Silica

Sulphur

Symphytum

Urtica urens

Veratrum album

STORING YOUR HOME KIT

All homeopathic remedies should be stored in a moderately cool, dry, dark place away from strong odors and temperature extremes. Products containing menthol and camphor (such as those discussed in "What to Avoid") can reduce or cancel the effectiveness of homeopathic remedies. Cabinets, closets, or drawers that have strong odors from perfumes, aromatic creams, or mothballs are *not* good places to store remedies. Find a neutral, odor-free place in your home for your remedies. When properly stored they will last indefinitely. Remedy bottles or tubes are stamped with an expiration date only because of a regulatory requirement. Remedies over one hundred years old have been known to be effective.

If you travel with homeopathic remedies, do not put them through an airport X-ray machine. This has been known to render them ineffective. Metal detectors, however, will generally not affect remedies.

A WORD ABOUT ARNICA MONTANA

The First Aid Remedy, *Arnica montana* is a truly wonderful and healing remedy. Many people have been introduced to and won over by homeopathy because of *Arnica*. It is so effective in a wide range of injury and trauma conditions that if you had to choose only one remedy for your first aid kit, *Arnica* would be it. Even when another remedy for an injury may be indicated but is not available, oftentimes *Arnica* can be given with benefit. When preparing your home remedy kit, I recommend that you include *Arnica* 30C as well as *Arnica* 200C. These are invaluable to have on hand in case of more serious trauma. For more details about *Arnica*, see Part 6.

USEFUL EXTERNAL APPLICATIONS

The following external applications will help soothe and heal a variety of ailments. They may be used alone or in conjunction with the appropriate internal remedy. Some of these products are formulated by a particular homeopathic manufacturer; they are indicated in parentheses. All others are available from a number of sources, some of which are listed in the "Internet Resources Directory."

Creams or ointments are oil and/or wax-based medicated applications. The emolliency helps to soothe and provide a protective moisture barrier.

Gels are water-based medicated applications, sometimes containing glycerin or a small amount of alcohol.

Lotions are tinctures that have been diluted with water. They are used for cleaning, bathing, or soaking an injured part.

Oils are pure medicinal plant oils, usually mixed with extender or vehicle oils, such as almond, jojoba, or peanut oil.

Tinctures are solutions made from a plant prepared in alcohol, usually sold in an amber dropper bottle. Not potentized, they are also called mother tinctures and are the substances from which many potentized remedies are made.

AESCULUS OINTMENT A soothing hemorrhoid ointment that may include *Hamamelis* and/or *Collinsonia*.

ARNICA CREAM OR OINTMENT Apply to bruises, sore muscles, sprains, strains, and any injury from overuse or blunt trauma. Apply to *unbroken skin only* (never to an open wound or cut, because it would cause a painful irritation). When applied early enough, *Arnica* can reverse the black and blue process in a very short time.

ARNICA OIL (Weleda) Excellent for the massage of sore, aching muscles and in strains and sprains; also provides an extra layer of protective warmth during cold weather.

BURN CARE GEL (Weleda) For burns, sunburn, insect bites and stings; contains *Arnica* and *Urtica urens*.

CALENDULA (*Marigold*) **BABY POWDER** For diaper rash and athlete's foot.

CALENDULA CREAM OR OINTMENT For scrapes, cuts, sores, and rashes.

CALENDULA SPRAY (Hyland's) A nonalcohol, glycerin-based juice that can be sprayed on tender skin directly without dilution.

CALENDULA TINCTURE For scrapes, cuts, sores, rashes, and as a mouthwash ingredient.

EUPHRASIA (*Eyebright*) **TINCTURE** For bathing the eye in the case of infection, inflammation, or injury.

HYPERCAL CREAM (Nelsons) A combination of *Hypericum* and *Calendula* that can be applied to scrapes, cuts, and sores, especially where there is much pain in areas rich in nerves, such as fingertips and toes.

HYPERICUM (*St. John's wort*) **TINCTURE** For cuts, wounds, or insect bites; sharp, shooting pains.

LEDUM (*Marsh Tea*) **TINCTURE** For puncture wounds, tick bites, or animal bites.

MULLEIN (*Verbascum*) **OIL** For earaches, especially recommended in households with young children. Sometimes sold as ear drops or ear oil drops, mullein oil often comes mixed with garlic, St. John's wort, or *Calendula* oil. Mullein oil is to be used only in earaches where there is no discharge.

RESCUE REMEDY A preparation made from five flower essences, for trauma or distress of any kind; provides broad-based emergency support, helping a person stay balanced and grounded during times of trauma, accident, or a wide range of acute emotional and physical crises. The drops may be taken directly under the tongue or diluted in water. Rescue Remedy may be used concurrently with another internal remedy, but avoid taking it at the same moment.

STING GEL (Nelsons) For insect bites and stings; a combination of remedies including *pyrethrum, Ledum, Arnica, Hypericum,* and others.

THUJA OINTMENT For use with fungal infections and warts.

TRAUMEEL OINTMENT (BHI) Also called Traumed, a combination of *Arnica* and other first aid remedies for sprains, sore joints, and muscles; for use with sports injuries, repetitive or overuse injuries, and trauma. Although this is not a classical homeopathic preparation, it can be applied in a wide range of first aid situations. Do not use on broken skin or open wounds.

URTICA URENS (*Stinging Nettle*) TINCTURE For insect bites and stings, burns, and sunburn.

KITCHEN REMEDIES

The following kitchen remedies can be helpful complements to homeopathic treatment. They may be used in conjunction with a homeopathic remedy, alone, or when a homeopathic remedy is either not available or not indicated.

Aloe vera gel—for burns and minor cuts and scrapes
Baking soda—for insect bites and mineral baths
Carrot—for ear compresses
Chamomile tea—for stomach upset and abdominal cramps
Charcoal powder capsules—for insect bites and poisoning
Epsom salts—for mineral baths for muscular aches and pains
Fresh ginger—for digestive complaints and respiratory congestion
Raw honey—for sore throats, hay fever prevention, as an
    antiseptic for burns
Ice pack—for injuries, swelling, bruises, insect bites
Lemon—for fever; preventive at the first sign of colds and flu
Onion—for ear compresses
Sage tea—for sore throats and hoarseness
Sea salt—for gargling and mineral baths

CREATING A HEALING ATMOSPHERE

While caring for yourself or others with homeopathy, it is worthwhile to consider any influences that may enhance or detract from the healing process. Factors such as the immediate environment, rest, and diet can affect how quickly and completely a person recovers. Good quality caregiving, whether applied to yourself or another, can help stimulate the healing process and ease suffering. When caring for someone who is ill or convalescing, keep in mind these suggestions:

IMMEDIATE ENVIRONMENT: Keep the bedroom clean, orderly, and dust free. Air the room periodically while the person is out of the room; fresh air is essential. Keep the room comfortably warm, at 68 to 72 degrees Fahrenheit. Supply ample fresh fluids at the bedside, as well as tissues and a wastebasket. A soothing environment for the senses will help the healing process. Fresh flowers can lift the spirits. If possible, avoid overstimulation with television and other electronic media, which can significantly interfere with the quality of rest.

REST AND SLEEP: Keep a regular sleep schedule when well, and get plenty of quiet rest when ill. Rest and sleep are vitally important for prevention and during illness. No medicine can replace the value of sound sleep. It is all too common that people "just don't have time" to get sick. Do allow for healing time. If homeopathy is new to you, you may be pleasantly surprised by how quickly you and your loved ones can recover from illness.

DIET: Illness is often a time of cleansing. It is therefore important to eat a simple, nourishing diet that does not overtax digestion. When we are ill common sense and lack of appetite often guide us away from rich or heavy foods. It is not unusual to completely lose one's appetite when sick; this is nature's way of helping us cleanse. Fresh, gently cooked vegetables, broth, and moderate amounts of whole grains are suggested during illness. Partial or complete fasting from solid food can be highly beneficial during many types of illnesses.

WARMTH: Essential in maintaining good health as well as during illness, warmth is a frequently overlooked aspect of prevention; too often one can look back and say, "If only I had been dressed more warmly." Children especially need warmth for proper development and maintenance of good health. Babies lose body heat rapidly through their proportionately larger heads and should wear pilot-type caps or bonnets throughout the year. Aside from looking cute, a cap protects the delicate membranes of the skull from sun, heat, cold, and air-conditioning while helping to prevent ear infections and other common illnesses. A thick cotton or wool undershirt, long-johns, or tights should be underwear staples in a child's daily wardrobe from fall through midspring in most climates. It is advisable for people of all ages to dress in several layers except in the hottest weather. During illness, even fever, provide adequate covering. Last but not least, warmth comes in the form of love and kindness, which certainly aid the healing process. As with homeopathic remedies, a small dose of these can make a big difference.

PART 3

HOMEOPATHIC FIRST AID

There are many first aid situations in which homeopathy is effective in alleviating pain and emotional distress while helping the body to heal itself. Homeopathy has an excellent track record with a wide variety of health emergencies and is fairly simple to use. Seeing how quickly a homeopathic remedy can give relief can be tremendously gratifying.

The highest priority in case of injury or accident is to keep a cool head (and a warm heart) and use commonsense first aid measures while seeking emergency medical care when necessary. Whether homeopathy is used at the outset or later in the healing process, a well-selected remedy can reduce pain significantly and speed up healing to a remarkable degree. In case you cannot administer a first aid remedy right away, remember that the correct remedy, even if given later, can be a big help.

In order to give the best first aid care, become familiar with the homeopathic first aid guidelines in this book before the need arises and learn and practice basic first aid measures. It is essential to know, for example, how to stop bleeding, attend to wounds, apply a bandage, and so on. I highly recommend getting an illustrated guide to emergency medical procedures; many good first aid manuals are available. Learning more advanced skills such as artificial respiration or CPR (cardiopulmonary resuscitation) is a big asset that can save a life. Consider taking a first aid course to get hands-on training. There is nothing like experience to make you a competent and confident provider of first aid.

Most first aid conditions have external causes and are generally not related to a person's susceptibility. There are less common instances, however, in which an injury could be related to a more serious internal problem, such as when a person injures her knee from falling as the result of a seizure or stroke. If you suspect such an underlying cause, of course a trip to the hospital is warranted. Give a dose or two of *Arnica* while riding to the emergency room.

However, prescribing for most first aid conditions is generally quite simple and straightforward. The symptoms have an urgency that will speak clearly and strongly. Because susceptibility is not a factor in the majority of cases, there will be fewer unique and individualizing symptoms. The remedies from which to choose will be limited to a smaller group known for success in treating specific conditions.

The following homeopathic recommendations are for acute, short-term first aid situations. Any injury or its resulting condition that has a tendency to show chronic effects over a prolonged period should be treated by a professional homeopath or other health care provider.

DOSAGE AND POTENCY FOR FIRST AID

The guidelines for first aid treatment are generally the same as those in "Selecting the Potency and Dosage." Do keep in mind that many first aid conditions have strong and acutely urgent symptoms; therefore you may need to repeat the remedy more frequently or use a higher potency than with a minor or gradually developing illness. Some first aid treatments have specific dosage recommendations. Unless otherwise noted, observe the following guidelines:

VERY SERIOUS CONDITIONS: Injuries that may be life threatening or require urgent attention and are often accompanied by severe pain or distress, for example, serious burns; back and head injuries; traumatic shock; poisonous insect or animal bites; unconsciousness; trauma with difficult breathing, serious bleeding or bruising, or internal injuries

Seek emergency medical care at once. While awaiting help or riding to the emergency room, give one dose every five to fifteen minutes, in the highest potency you are confident using or have available: 6C, 12C, or 30C. *Arnica* 200C may be given in many of these conditions. Repeat as needed according to the severity *until symptoms lessen:* every one to three hours as the condition improves, and thereafter three to four times per day for three days.

MODERATELY SERIOUS CONDITIONS: Symptoms that are serious but not life threatening, for example, bad sprains, fractures, moderately bleeding wounds, second-degree burns

Give one dose of 12C or 30C frequently (every five to thirty minutes) for the first two or three doses, then less often (every one to three hours) as symptoms improve.

LESS SERIOUS CONDITIONS: Symptoms accompanied by moderate discomfort or pain, for example, stiff or sore muscles from overexertion, minor sprains, bruises, and cuts

Give one dose three or four times per day. Use 6C or 12C, more or less often according to severity of symptoms. A 30C potency may be given if you feel more certain about the remedy choice, or if the lower potencies are not on hand.

Remember: Give only *one* remedy at a time. Stop giving the remedy *when there is improvement,* and repeat it only as needed.

FIRST AID CONDITIONS

BACK INJURIES AND BACKACHE

Whether from lifting, straining, overexertion, or a fall or a blow, acute back pain can be one of the most incapacitating common ailments. Homeopathy will provide welcome relief for many acute back complaints, although some injuries may require additional support with physical therapy or other intervention. Back pain that recurs frequently needs constitutional homeopathic treatment.

For a serious back injury professional care is a must. In case of a severe injury, do not move the person. Call 911 and give *Arnica* 30C every ten minutes until emergency help arrives; give *Arnica* 200C every ten minutes instead if it is available, especially if there are multiple serious injuries including any of the following: head injury, significant bruising or bleeding, broken bones, or unconsciousness, or if you suspect internal injuries.

When a back injury occurs, select one of these homeopathic remedies and give at frequent intervals until the severity of the symptoms lessens. Then give it less often as symptoms improve.

ARNICA MONTANA

- The primary remedy for back injuries

- Strains from lifting or twisting; trauma from a fall or blow

- Bruised, aching, sore feeling; the bed feels too hard

- Aversion to being touched

- After the initial shock, *Arnica* may be followed by another remedy if needed

BRYONIA ALBA

- Much aching and stiffness; sharp pains from movement

- Worse from the slightest movement or jarring; must keep still

- Better from steady pressure or lying on painful area

- May be irritable and wants to be left alone

HYPERICUM

- Injuries from a fall or blow

- Injuries, including fracture, especially to the spine or tailbone (coccyx)

- Spinal injuries where there is much sharp, shooting pain

- Sharp nerve pains that extend up the spine or down the leg

- Worse from raising arms or from movement

RHUS TOXICODENDRON

- Injuries from straining, lifting, or overexertion, especially to the lower back

- Much pain, stiffness, and restlessness

- Worse from prolonged sitting or resting, from first movements after rest, and from cold

- Better from continued gentle motion, rubbing, firm pressure, and warmth

COMMONSENSE MEASURES

- Adequate rest is absolutely essential following a back injury. Ask to what degree freedom of movement is limited and how much pain there is. Let the answers guide the recovery period.

- During the first twenty-four to forty-eight hours, you may apply an ice pack to the affected area to reduce swelling and inflammation.

- Afterward a warm compress or a soak in a warm bath can relieve soreness, stiffness, and knotted muscles. To further ease discomfort you may add to the bath 1 cup of Epsom salts or ½ cup each of baking soda and sea salt.

- Apply *Arnica* cream or Traumed ointment three times a day, or massage with *Arnica* oil to complement the internal remedy. Ease back into normal activity gently.

SEEK PROFESSIONAL HELP

- If there is difficulty moving legs or if they feel numb

- If back pain is accompanied by fever, nausea, or vomiting (when it's not influenza)

- If a back injury results in loss of bowel or bladder control, or if urine looks bloody

- If symptoms are not improving steadily

BLEEDING

A well-selected homeopathic remedy can help stop bleeding quickly and effectively in many first aid situations. Give one of the following remedies, according to the severity of the condition, every ten to thirty minutes. Stop when there is improvement, and repeat the remedy only as needed. For more information on nosebleeds, see Part 5.

ACONITE
- Marked anxiety, restlessness, and fear with bleeding

ARNICA MONTANA
- Shock and trauma with bleeding wounds; with bruising
- Will help stop both internal and external bleeding

FERRUM PHOSPHORICUM
- Bleeding head wounds, after *Arnica* has been given

HAMAMELIS
- Profuse bleeding of wounds or cuts
- If *Arnica* did not stop the bleeding
- Useful in nosebleeds (*Phosphorus*)

IPECACUANHA
- Injuries with bright red blood; nosebleeds
- Bleeding accompanied by nausea, labored breathing, or faintness

PHOSPHORUS
- Primary remedy (along with *Hamamelis*) for nosebleeds with bright red blood
- Thirst for ice water
- Any bleeding wound in a person who has many *Phosphorus* characteristics (see Part 6)

COMMONSENSE MEASURES

- Apply pressure and ice according to standard first aid procedure.

- Keep the person quiet and resting.

SEEK PROFESSIONAL HELP

- If bleeding is severe or if none of the previous suggestions is helping

- At once if you suspect internal bleeding after an injury. If the pulse rate is increased after external bleeding has been stopped, internal bleeding is likely.

BLISTERS

Most blisters are caused by either friction or a burn. Although it is tempting, try not to burst blisters. This will invite infection. Protect them with a bandage and they will recede in time.

COMMONSENSE MEASURES

- If blisters do break, prepare a healing lotion by combining equal parts *Hypericum* and *Calendula* tinctures, diluted in three times as much water (1:3 = 6 drops of each tincture added to 36 drops of water). Apply this solution with a gauze pad two or three times per day. Alternatively you may use *Calendula* spray (a non-alcohol, glycerin-based solution) directly on blisters, or apply Hypercal cream.

- Burst blisters should remain covered until they start to dry up. Allow them to finish healing uncovered. To treat blisters caused by poison oak or ivy, chicken pox, or burns, see those sections.

SEEK PROFESSIONAL HELP

- If blisters or the surrounding area becomes extremely painful or infected

BRUISES

Bruises are caused by a fall or blow that breaks the blood vessels under the skin, resulting in black and blue discoloration. For bruising or the likelihood of bruising following any accident or trauma, the remedy is *Arnica*. Superficial bruises that cause mild pain may be treated with *Arnica* cream alone. Do not hesitate, though, to give *Arnica* internally when there is marked pain or distress from shock, or to prevent bruising immediately following an injury. *Arnica* is also helpful in treating aching and soreness caused by overexertion or sports injuries when there is a generalized bruised feeling.

ARNICA MONTANA

- Bruises caused by a fall or blow; any type of accident or injury

- Aching, soreness, aversion to being touched

HYPERICUM

- Injuries to areas rich in nerves: spine, fingers, genitals

- Crushing injuries to fingertips or toes

- Marked sharp, shooting pains

Give *Arnica* in any potency, depending on the severity of the injury. Give it at more frequent intervals until symptoms lessen. If swelling is anticipated, ice may also be applied. *Hypericum* may be given at the outset or shortly after *Arnica* when its use is indicated.

SEEK PROFESSIONAL HELP

- If bruising is severe, extensive, or is indicative of deeper internal injury

BURNS

Many burns can be successfully treated with homeopathy. Even with serious burns for which medical care must be sought, homeopathy can bring swift pain relief, speed the healing process, and prevent excessive blistering or scarring. It is important to assess the severity of a burn:

- A first-degree burn leaves the skin reddened and painful without blistering.

- A second-degree burn causes blistering in addition to redness and pain.

- A third-degree burn has penetrated deeper layers of the skin and may be painless because of nerve damage. The severely burned area may appear either white or charred black. Third-degree burns always require immediate medical attention.

APIS MELLIFICA
- Minor burns, relieved by cold applications
- Marked heat, redness, swelling, and stinging pain

Give *Apis* 6C or 12C every fifteen minutes for three or four doses. Repeat if necessary, less often as symptoms improve.

ARNICA MONTANA
- For the shock of second- or third-degree burns

Arnica may be given as a single dose immediately following a second- or third-degree burn, *before giving Cantharis or Arsenicum,* to alleviate shock. *Arnica* may also be given repeatedly to treat shock in third-degree burns if this symptom is uppermost. (See "Shock.")

ARSENICUM ALBUM

- Serious second- or third-degree burns

- Severe burning pain

- Anxiety, fear, and restlessness

- Marked chilliness and weakness

- Aversion to cold applications, desire to wrap up warmly

Give *Arsenicum* 12C or 30C every fifteen minutes for three or four doses. Repeat if necessary, less often as symptoms improve.

CANTHARIS

- Serious burns, primary remedy in second- and third-degree burns

- Severely painful burns, better from cold applications

- Burns with blisters

- Chemical burns

- Marked restlessness may be present with burning pain

Cantharis is highly effective in relieving painful and serious burns and, if given soon enough, will prevent blister formation. Give 12C or 30C every fifteen minutes for three or four doses. Repeat if necessary, less often as symptoms improve.

CARBOLIC ACID

- Chemical burns

- Later stages of healing in extensive burns

For later stages of healing, give *Carbolic acid* 12C once daily for up to two weeks. Discontinue as soon as there is marked improvement.

CAUSTICUM

- Burns that have left painful or poorly healed scars, even from long ago

- Recent burns that fail to heal well; cracking and ulceration

Sometimes, despite diligent care, a serious burn may not heal satisfactorily. *Causticum* is excellent for poorly healed burns. Give *Causticum* 12C or 30C three times per day for up to three days.

PHOSPHORUS

- Electrical burns

Give *Phosphorus* 12C or 30C three times a day for up to three days following an electrical burn.

URTICA URENS

- Primary remedy for first-degree burns and scalds

- Burns from hot water, sunburns

- Minor burns without blistering; sensation of burning and itching combined

Urtica urens, made from stinging nettle, will bring great relief in painful burns and scalds. Give 6C or 12C right away, every fifteen minutes for three or four doses. This dosage should be sufficient to quell most of the pain.

COMMONSENSE MEASURES

- Remove a burn victim from any further risk of harm.

- For third-degree burns, do not apply any external treatments, call 911, and encourage but do not force the person to drink water. Give the appropriate internal remedy.

- Quickly remove any clothing from burned areas. Liquid burns may cause clothing to stick to the skin. Carefully cut around clothing to expose as much of the burn as you can.

- In first- and second-degree burns, immerse the burned part in cool water for at least five minutes. Adding a few drops of *Urtica urens* or *Hypericum* tincture to the water beforehand will help reduce pain and prevent blisters.

- After the initial cooling of the burn, you may use the homeopathic application of small doses of heat. Blistering, burning pains, scarring, and overall healing time have been proven to be substantially minimized with homeopathic heat treatment in comparison with similar burns treated only with cold. Following a burn to the hand, for example, pass it near a heat source (such as a stove) just until the heat stings a little. Quickly withdraw the hand and repeat. Do this rhythmically for a minute or so until the pain subsides. You will be surprised at how fast it works. This homeopathic method of "taking a hair of the dog that bit you" or "fighting fire with fire" is well known among European chefs. Continue with the following steps as needed. (Note: Heat treatment is not appropriate for severe second- and third-degree burns.)

- Apply *Urtica urens* lotion, ¼ teaspoon of the tincture mixed with ½ cup clean water. A strip of gauze or linen cloth soaked in the solution may be applied to keep the burn moist until smarting is reduced. Burn care gel may be applied if the skin is unbroken.

- Where blisters have broken, *Calendula* lotion or spray may be applied to prevent infection and scarring. Use three or four times per day to speed healing. *Calendula* cream may be applied but only after the burn has cooled. A fresh burn should never be treated with anything that contains grease or oil—this will only "fry" the burn and cause greater suffering.

- *Aloe vera* gel is also a very soothing, healing, and convenient application for many types of burns. An aloe plant kept on your kitchen windowsill is quite handy: just break off a leaf of the plant and squeeze out the gel onto a burn. *Aloe*, like *Calendula*, is excellent for preventing scarring in burns and other wounds.

- Sunburns may be sprayed with *Urtica urens* lotion. Apply the solution with a spray bottle for refreshing relief.

- Chemical burns must be washed thoroughly under cold running water.

- It should go without saying that an ounce of prevention is worth a pound of cure; many burns are preventable, and it is worth assessing the risk factors in your home. Check for faulty electrical appliances, keep matches and fuels away from curious little hands, and do not smoke in bed or anywhere you are likely to fall asleep. Working smoke alarms and a fire extinguisher are musts in every home.

SEEK PROFESSIONAL HELP

- For any third-degree burn call 911 or go to the emergency room immediately.

- For second-degree burns that occur to any of the following areas: eyes, ears, face, genitals, hands, or feet

- If a burn covers an area larger than your hand

- Electrical burns

- Chemical burns, unless very mild

CUTS AND SCRAPES

CALENDULA

- Wonderful external treatment for cuts, scrapes, and shallow wounds

HYPERICUM

- Take internally for painful cuts, especially to the fingers or toes, or any part that is rich in nerves.

- Cuts with sharp or shooting pain.

In addition, *Hypericum* or *Hypercal* ointment may be applied externally for painful cuts.

COMMONSENSE MEASURES

- Clean the affected area by washing it with *Calendula* lotion (about 15 drops of mother tincture in 4 ounces of water). Alternatively, rinse with water, apply *Calendula* spray, and gently pat dry. Make sure you have removed gravel, dirt, or other foreign material. Next apply *Calendula* ointment and cover with a bandage; reapply the dressing as needed. *Calendula* is so effective in closing wounds that it should not be applied to deeper ones unless they are absolutely clean, for risk of enclosing an infection. Apply diluted *Hypericum* tincture or Hypercal ointment to deeper cuts or where there is much sharp, shooting pain. Give *Hypericum* pellets internally if needed for pain. (To treat deeper wounds, see "Puncture Wounds and Animal Bites.")

DROWNING

Reviving a drowning person requires quick action. Call 911 immediately and give artificial respiration and/or CPR according to the guidelines in a standard first aid manual. Persist in your efforts until help arrives. Give one of the following remedies every five minutes until improvement is seen. If possible, crush the pellets to a powder first and place the remedy between the cheek and lower gums. Give the alternate remedy if there is no change after three doses.

ANTIMONIUM TARTARICUM

- First remedy to consider for drowning

- The person is blue with clammy skin

- Rattling, wet respiration

- Face may be sunken and gaunt

CARBO VEGETABILIS

- Second remedy to consider for drowning

- The person is blue and cold, with icy hands and feet

- Face may be puffy, bloated, or mottled

SEEK PROFESSIONAL HELP

- Always call 911 immediately.

- A person who recovers from drowning must always be checked by a doctor because of the risk of respiratory infection.

EYE INJURIES

A simple black eye or minor scratch to the cornea may be treated at home; however, any injury to the eye that causes severe swelling, pain, or impaired vision merits prompt medical attention. In such cases give the appropriate remedy on the way to the doctor's office or emergency room. The following remedies can help relieve pain and distress, and promote healing of the delicate tissues of the eye.

ACONITE

- First remedy to consider immediately after eye injury

- Eye injury accompanied by fear, anxiety, and restlessness

- Abrasion to the cornea from foreign objects, sand, or dust

- Black eye, when trauma to the eyeball is minor

Aconite is often referred to as the *Arnica* of the eye and can provide great relief when given as soon after the injury as possible. *Aconite* may be followed by one of the following remedies to continue the healing process. Often one to three doses of *Aconite* 30C every fifteen minutes are enough to reduce initial distress and pain. Repeat if needed, or follow with another remedy.

ARNICA MONTANA

- Blunt trauma to the eye

- Primary remedy for a black eye

- Bloodshot eye caused by injury

Arnica is the first general remedy for the shock of an eye injury and often follows *Aconite*. *Arnica* will help absorb the blood that causes bruising and reddening of the eye, and will also reduce swelling and pain. Following the injury give *Arnica* 30C every fifteen to thirty minutes for three or four doses, then less often with continued improvement. Thereafter *Arnica* may be given three or four times a day for up to one week.

LEDUM PALUSTRE

- Black eye

- When pain, bruising, and swelling continue after *Arnica*

- Marked relief when cold is applied

Ledum is often indicated when the black and blue has begun to turn green and yellow. Give *Ledum* 12C or 30C two or three times per day as needed for up to one week.

SYMPHYTUM

- On a par with *Arnica* after a blow to the eye from a blunt object, such as a baseball

- Injuries to bones surrounding the eye

- Lingering eye injuries, where bruised pain remains after *Arnica*

Symphytum is known for its excellence in both trauma to the eyeball and bone injuries from blunt objects. Give *Symphytum* every fifteen to thirty minutes for three or four doses, then less often with improvement. Thereafter *Symphytum* may be given three or four times per day for up to one week.

COMMONSENSE MEASURES

- For a mild scratch on the cornea caused by sand, dirt, or other foreign matter, flush the eye thoroughly with *Hypericum* and *Calendula* lotion: Add 2 drops of each mother tincture to 2 ounces of either distilled water or sterile saline solution. This will soothe the injury and may dislodge the material. If the eye is still painful after removal of the object, bathe it with *Euphrasia* lotion, prepared in the same manner as just described. If the object cannot be removed, cover the eye with a clean cloth and get prompt medical attention.

- For a black eye, apply an ice pack or a bag of frozen peas to reduce swelling.

- *Calendula* lotion or ointment may be applied to cuts or abrasions around the eye.

- *Arnica* ointment may be applied to bruised and swollen areas surrounding the eye; however, do not apply *Arnica* to any skin that is broken, nor should any *Arnica* product go directly in the eye.

SEEK PROFESSIONAL HELP

- If foreign material cannot be flushed from the eye

- If glass or splinters are lodged in the eye

- If vision is blurred or impaired in any way

- If there is marked bleeding within the eyeball or externally

- If chemicals have gotten into the eye. Flush with running water until help is available.

FAINTING

Simple fainting may be caused by a myriad of factors; emotional upset, fright, exhaustion, the sight of blood, or being in a hot, stuffy room are a few examples. The cause of fainting may be an underlying illness. Fainting that lasts more than several minutes can be a sign of another serious condition, such as internal bleeding. If the immediate cause of a simple faint is known, give one of the following remedies every five or ten minutes for up to six doses.

ACONITE
- Fainting from fright

CARBO VEGETABILIS
- Fainting or collapse from weakness, exhaustion, lack of air, or any unknown cause

- With air hunger, cold breath; clammy or bluish skin

CHAMOMILLA
- Fainting from severe pain

CHINA
- Fainting from loss of blood, such as from a bleeding wound or heavy menstruation

COFFEA CRUDA
• Fainting from overexcitement or surprise

HEPAR SULPHURIS
• Fainting from minor pain

IGNATIA AMARA
• Fainting from intense emotion or hysteria

NUX VOMICA
• Fainting from the sight of blood

• Fainting from smelling strong odors

PULSATILLA
• Fainting from being in hot, stuffy surroundings

SILICA
• Fainting from the sight of needles

COMMONSENSE MEASURES
• Simple fainting rarely lasts more than a few moments. Make the person comfortable. Loosen any clothing that restricts breathing, and make sure the surroundings give adequate fresh air. As the person comes around, offer reassurance and a drink of water to which a few drops of Rescue Remedy have been added. Encourage breathing deeply. People who are prone to fainting will benefit from constitutional homeopathic treatment.

SEEK PROFESSIONAL HELP
• If fainting lasts more than a few minutes, seek emergency care at once.

FRACTURED BONES

A fracture occurs when a bone is either cracked or broken through. In both cases there is pain, swelling, and often great difficulty moving the injured part. Whether a remedy is given during the first few hours, days, or later on, homeopathic treatment can be highly effective in reducing pain and promoting healing of broken bones.

ARNICA MONTANA
- First remedy for initial shock, pain, bruising, and swelling of fractures

Depending on the severity of the injury and pain, give *Arnica* immediately following the injury, one or two doses within the first hour. Afterward *Arnica* may be given every one to three hours, less often over the next few days as needed. Consider the following remedies as well after the initial shock has passed.

BRYONIA ALBA
- Broken or cracked ribs

- Pain from the slightest movement, even breathing

Give *Bryonia* every two to four hours during the day or two after the initial trauma, less often as needed thereafter.

CALCAREA PHOSPHORICA
- Slow-to-heal fractures or old fractures where pain remains

- Pain is worse during cold weather

- Especially for elderly people

- In people with a history of weak or brittle bones or teeth

After *Arnica* has been given for the initial phase, give *Calcarea phosphorica* 6X or 6C, three times per day over a two- to four-week period as needed for slow-healing fractures or individuals with weakened bones.

EUPATORIUM PERFOLIATUM

- Often follows *Arnica*

- During the initial phase of healing from a fracture

- When a deep aching pain predominates over bruising or swelling

Eupatorium comes from a North American plant commonly called boneset because of its traditional use in the healing of broken bones. Give *Eupatorium* every two to four hours during the first few days, less often as needed thereafter.

HYPERICUM

- Crushed bones, especially fingers and toes

- Sharp, shooting nerve pains

- Primary remedy in compound fractures (where the broken bone is exposed through a wound in the skin)

Give *Hypericum* 12C or 30C shortly after the injury as you would *Arnica*, at frequent intervals during the first twenty-four hours. Repeat three times per day for up to one week as needed. Another remedy such as *Symphytum* may be necessary to complete healing.

SYMPHYTUM

- Often follows *Arnica*; acts quickly to mend fractures

- The bone must be set properly before giving *Symphytum*

- Excellent for bones that are slow to heal

Symphytum, derived from the common plant comfrey, is traditionally called knitbone for its bone-mending abilities. Give 12C or 30C soon after the injury as you would *Arnica*. For later stages of healing, give *Symphytum* 6X or 6C, three times per day over a two- to four-week period as needed for slow-healing fractures.

COMMONSENSE MEASURES

- If you suspect a fracture, visit a doctor; an X ray may be necessary to confirm that a fracture has occurred. All fractures must be evaluated by a skilled professional.

- Do not try to move the injured part if you suspect it is broken.

- Attend to any cuts or wounds that may have accompanied the fracture while you wait for help. Give reassurance and a few drops of Rescue Remedy if there is distress.

SEEK PROFESSIONAL HELP

- If you suspect that a fracture has occurred

- If there is marked bleeding or bruising beneath the skin

- If an injured part is numb, severely painful, or cannot be used

HEAD INJURIES AND WHIPLASH

No one goes through life without a good bang on the head once in a while. Most common head injuries amount to a bruising or a goose-egg lump and do not constitute cause for alarm. However, deeper injury to the skull or brain can occur, and in some instances this may not be apparent for up to twenty-four hours. Watch for complications during the forty-eight hours following the injury. Anyone who suffers a serious blow to the head or neck should receive immediate medical attention. In such a case give the appropriate internal remedy on the way to the doctor or emergency room.

ARNICA MONTANA

- The primary remedy for a blow to the head

- Person may say he is well when he is not

As always, *Arnica* is the remedy of choice for trauma. It will relieve pain and shock as well as swelling, bruising, and bleeding. Give *Arnica* frequently at first, every fifteen minutes to one hour depending on severity, less often as symptoms improve. *Arnica* may be given three or four times per day as long as symptoms are present, for up to seven days.

HYPERICUM

- Damage to the spine, neck, or nerves following a head injury

- Head and neck injuries with sharp, shooting pain

- Convulsions caused by head injury

- Whiplash

Hypericum is helpful in cases of whiplash or nerve pains in the neck associated with head injury. Give as needed, three times per day for up to seven days.

NATRUM SULPHURICUM

- Pain that persists after head injury, even years later

- The person has never felt well since a head injury

- Mental, emotional, or personality changes after a head injury

After *Arnica* has been given, consider *Natrum sulphuricum* when a person does not fully recover from a head injury or feels somehow changed for the worse since the event. If after the first week there is depression, confusion, or mistakes in speaking, writing, or reading,

Natrum sulphuricum 12C may be given once daily for several weeks until improvement occurs. Seek professional advice for these types of difficulties.

COMMONSENSE MEASURES

- Apply an ice pack to an uncomplicated bang on the head, where no signs of deeper trauma are present. Attend to any external wounds. With a concussion, keep the person awake until he or she can be evaluated by a professional health care provider. Encourage periods of rest and quiet each day until fully recovered.

SEEK PROFESSIONAL HELP

Immediate medical care should be sought:

- After any severe head injury

- If there is significant pain moving the head or neck

- If there are any lapses or changes in consciousness within forty-eight hours of the injury

- If there is confusion, loss of memory, restlessness, marked drowsiness or weakness, slurred speech, twitching, unusual eye movements, or visual disturbance

- If the pupils have become unequal in size

- If changes in mental, emotional, or physical well-being persist

- If there are convulsions

- If there is blood or clear fluid coming from the ears or nose

- If there is repeated vomiting after the first two hours

HEAT EXHAUSTION AND SUNSTROKE

Heat exhaustion (or heat prostration) is caused by prolonged exposure to hot weather combined with dehydration resulting from perspiration, lack of water intake, or excessive use of alcohol. Symptoms usually develop gradually, with weakness, dizziness, and confusion, and the skin becomes pale, cold, and sweaty. There may also be difficulty breathing, nausea, and muscle cramps. Sunstroke (heatstroke) is a more serious condition, in which the body's cooling abilities stop functioning because of overheating. Sunstroke and heat exhaustion share some symptoms, except that sunstroke symptoms may develop more rapidly. In sunstroke the skin is hot, dry, and red, with fever and throbbing headache. Convulsions and unconsciousness may occur. Sunstroke can be life threatening. Seek emergency care at once if symptoms of sunstroke are present, and give the appropriate remedy while awaiting help. Homeopathic medicines can be highly effective for these conditions. Even if the person is markedly improved after the remedy, however, medical evaluation is recommended.

Select one of the following remedies, and give one dose every fifteen to thirty minutes, depending on the severity of symptoms. Repeat until there is improvement, then less often as needed. If after three doses there is no improvement, give a different remedy.

BELLADONNA

- Dry, hot, burning skin; fever may be present

- Severe throbbing headache, reddened face

- Dilated pupils, sensitivity to light

- Pulsating pain in head made worse by light, noise, jarring

- Stupor or delirium

- Better from bending head backward

CARBO VEGETABILIS

- Weakness, fainting, or collapse from exposure to heat and sun

- Cold, clammy skin

- Nausea and diarrhea

- Marked air hunger, must have cool air or be fanned

CUPRUM METALLICUM

- Severe cramping or jerking muscles

- Similar to *Veratrum album*, though less cold

GLONOINE

- Very similar to *Belladonna*, except

- Less burning of the skin

- Violent bursting pain in head

- Dizzy and drowsy

- Worse from bending head backward

NATRUM CARBONICUM

- Marked weakness from exposure to the sun the main symptom

- Headache, faintness, dizziness, or confusion

- Nausea or diarrhea may be present

VERATRUM ALBUM

- Profuse, clammy sweat with pale skin

- Marked coldness, especially of hands and feet

- Tremendous weakness

- Collapse or fainting may occur

- Nausea and vomiting

COMMONSENSE MEASURES
- Cool the person as quickly as possible. Have her lie down in the shade or a cool room and apply cold cloths to the head and body. If the temperature is elevated, immerse her in a cool bath, adding cold water as the bathwater becomes warm. Using very cold water initially may shock the person further; ease into it with care. Have her drink a glass of water with ½ teaspoon of salt added; repeat every thirty minutes over the next several hours. Rub the legs vigorously to promote circulation. If the person is unconscious, treat as you would for shock (see "Shock") and get immediate medical attention.

- Prevent heat exhaustion and sunstroke by drinking plenty of fluids, limiting exposure to the sun, and avoiding the use of alcohol in hot weather. Following heat exhaustion or sunstroke, precautions must be taken to prevent recurrence. Be sure to cover the head and use sunblock.

SEEK PROFESSIONAL HELP
- Immediately if you suspect sunstroke

- If fever is present and rising

- If there is fainting, unconsciousness, or convulsions

- If symptoms do not improve within one hour

INSECT BITES AND STINGS

Common insect bites and stings can be quite painful and occasionally can cause serious reactions. Fortunately, most insect bites produce a reaction that does not spread beyond the site of the sting. Whether the bite is from a mosquito, bee, wasp, common spider (or even a jellyfish), the circumscribed area of swelling, pain, itching, or redness shows that the body's natural defenses are at work, preventing the venom from affecting other areas.

Though less common, systemic reactions to bites and stings do occur. These symptoms range from the spreading of hives or other rash over a larger area to difficult breathing and wheezing, and loss of consciousness. Homeopathy can be effective in treating the full spectrum of reactions; however, emergency medical care must be sought in the more severe cases.

In an insect bite with mild to moderate symptoms, the suggested topical treatments may suffice. When an internal remedy is needed, select the one that most closely suits the condition, and give one dose every ten or fifteen minutes for two or three doses, less frequently as symptoms improve. If the localized reaction to the bite is intense, such as rapid swelling or extreme pain, give one dose of 30C every five or ten minutes until there is improvement. Repeat at less frequent intervals as symptoms continue to improve.

Bites from poisonous arachnids such as black widow spiders, tarantulas, or scorpions are more serious and often require immediate medical attention. While awaiting help apply an ice pack to slow the spread of the venom. You may also apply a poultice of activated charcoal to help draw out the venom.

For all types of bites, give one of the following remedies at five- to fifteen-minute intervals, depending on the severity of symptoms. Give less often as condition improves.

APIS MELLIFICA

- The second remedy to consider for a bite or sting

- Burning, stinging pain, with marked redness and puffy swelling

- Sensation of heat in the bitten part (opposite *Ledum*)

- Localized pain worse near heat, better from cold applications

- First remedy to consider when hives appear after a bite or sting

CARBOLIC ACID
- Weakness, faintness, and collapse

- Face is dusky red but can be pale around mouth and nose

- Shallow, difficult breathing

- The person may have an unusually acute sense of smell

LACHESIS
- Much purple discoloration and bruising around the bite

- Oozing of dark blood

LEDUM PALUSTRE
- The first remedy to consider for any insect bite or sting

- When no differentiating symptoms are present

- Stinging and prickling pain, with redness and swelling

- The bitten part may feel cold yet is relieved by cold applications

URTICA URENS
- Especially when burning, stinging, and itching are present in combination

- Second remedy (after *Apis*) to consider when hives appear after a bite or sting

COMMONSENSE MEASURES
- For prevention of stings and bites use insect repellent, preferably one without DEET or other chemical pesticides. Many natural repellents are available from health food stores and camping outfitters.

- In the case of a wasp, hornet, or bee sting, remove the stinger as soon as possible with tweezers or flick it off. (Take care not to squeeze the stinger; doing so can release more venom.) Apply sting gel, *Ledum* tincture, or burn care gel to soothe the area. If none of these is available, choose from the following topical treatments: Apply a baking soda paste (just baking soda and water) or a dab of mud; these will soothe the pain and also draw out the venom. Applying honey can also soothe a sting. Applying an ice pack to the area will slow the venom from spreading, reduce swelling, and relieve pain.

- Mosquito bites are seldom as painful as wasp or bee stings but can be maddeningly itchy and uncomfortable. Apply either sting gel or *Ledum* tincture. Especially itchy bites may respond well to burn care gel or *Urtica urens* tincture.

Some people, especially children, can be more susceptible to mosquito bites. If your child is prone to getting them, *Ledum* pellets may be given as a preventive: Give two or three doses during the twenty-four hours before likely exposure and up to three more doses during the first day. This is a short-term measure that should not be used habitually. The best means of achieving lasting results is constitutional homeopathic treatment.

- Tick bites are usually not too painful and can sometimes go unnoticed. Since Lyme disease has become an increasing problem, take the necessary precautions if you are visiting a tick-infested area.

In case of tick bite, saturate the site of the embedded tick (and the tick itself) with rubbing alcohol. This relaxes the tick (gets it drunk) and makes removal easier. Special tick tweezers will most often remove a tick effectively and completely. It can be very difficult to remove a tenacious tick with conventional tweezers, but applying alcohol does help. Next, apply Hypercal or *Calendula* cream. As an extra precaution with tick bites that occur in Lyme tick regions, bathe the area with *Ledum* tincture before applying cream, and give *Ledum*

30C internally three times per day for three days. Symptoms of Lyme disease must be evaluated by a health care professional. For further information on the symptoms and treatment of Lyme disease, contact the Lyme Disease Foundation, Inc., at www.lyme.org or the Lyme Disease Network at www.lymenet.org.

SEEK PROFESSIONAL HELP

- If there is difficulty breathing, marked weakness, or collapse

- If there is severe or rapid swelling

- If there is a history of severe reactions

- If there is a sting or swelling inside the mouth or throat

- If you suspect the bite is from a highly poisonous insect or arachnid

PUNCTURE WOUNDS AND ANIMAL BITES

Puncture wounds carry a greater risk of infection than shallow wounds because dirt, foreign material, and germs can be pushed deep into the body. The greatest danger is tetanus. Homeopathic remedies used externally and taken internally can minimize the risk of tetanus and infection while bringing pain relief and rapid healing. An animal bite is a type of puncture wound. The animal's saliva can carry an even greater risk of infection, including in some cases rabies. The most common carriers of rabies are wild raccoons, foxes, skunks, squirrels, and bats. Proper care of any puncture wound is essential. When rabies is a possibility, medical care must be sought immediately.

HYPERICUM

- Puncture wounds

- Animal and human bites

- Especially with sharp shooting pains

- If red streaks are present

Hypericum is quite helpful for puncture wounds, especially those that involve the nerves. Sharp, shooting pains are an indication, as well as the appearance of red streaks along the injured part. If either of these is present after giving *Ledum*, *Hypericum* will bring relief. Give one dose of *Hypericum* 12C or 30C every thirty minutes to one hour for two or three doses. Thereafter repeat every three or four hours, less often as there is improvement. As a preventive for tetanus, either *Ledum* or *Hypericum* 12C may be taken twice daily for ten days.

LEDUM PALUSTRE

- Primary remedy for a puncture wound from a nail, tack, wire, thorn, or similar object

- Primary remedy for animal or human bites

- Wound may feel cold to the touch, and feels better from cold applications

Ledum is a wonderful remedy for any puncture to the skin. *Ledum* will prevent infection and aid the body in healing the wound. Give *Ledum* 12C or 30C every thirty minutes to one hour for two or three doses. Repeat every four to six hours as needed, less often when there is improvement.

COMMONSENSE MEASURES

- Allow the puncture wound to bleed freely as long as possible to help eliminate any contaminating material. Gently squeeze around the wound if necessary. If bleeding is excessive, apply a cloth dressing soaked in *Hypericum* lotion, using gentle pressure.

- Cleanse the wound with soap and water, and soak in *Hypericum* lotion (15 drops tincture in 4 ounces of warm water) for ten or fifteen minutes. Alternatively, *Ledum* lotion may be used in this manner. Afterward cover the wound with a bandage. Soaking should be repeated several times a day while there is pain. *Calendula* in any form may be applied regularly once the interior of the wound is healing well and is beginning to close; *Calendula* is also excellent to help minimize scarring.

SEEK PROFESSIONAL HELP

- Immediately if there is a possibility of rabies from an animal bite

- If a puncture is very deep or dirty

- If a human bite punctures the skin

- If a puncture remains severely painful, becomes swollen or inflamed, or discharges pus

- If you are worried about tetanus. Among homeopaths, *Hypericum* and *Ledum* are known to be tetanus preventives, but they are not guarantees against the condition. Seek advice from an experienced homeopath or other health care provider about your particular condition. If you choose to have a tetanus injection, these remedies will still support the healing process.

SHOCK

There is an element of shock in any injury. Even when you bump your head, the breath catches, the pulse increases, and there may be a moment of panic. Greater degrees of shock will be seen in more serious trauma. In true shock the stress of an injury reduces blood flow and affects the functioning of the nervous system. Symptoms of shock include weakness; pale, cold, clammy skin; rapid pulse; and shallow breathing; there may also be fearfulness, restlessness, confusion, stupor, or unconsciousness. In serious injuries, such as major head trauma or severe burns, treatment for shock is vitally important. *Shock always requires emergency medical care.*

ACONITE

- Great restlessness and anxiety

- Great fearfulness; fear of death or impending doom

Aconite is most helpful when the primary reaction to an injury is emotional shock. *Aconite* will quickly calm this agitated and fearful state. Give *Aconite* 30C every fifteen to thirty minutes for three doses, less often as symptoms improve. In severe cases *Aconite* 200C may be given. Once the *Aconite* state has passed, select another remedy suited for the specific injury or condition.

ARNICA MONTANA

- The primary remedy for shock from any injury

Arnica will help stabilize the person and promote healing. Give *Arnica* 30C every fifteen to thirty minutes for three doses, less often as symptoms improve. In severe shock *Arnica* 200C may be given.

CARBO VEGETABILIS

- Weakness, coldness, and/or collapse prominent

- Air hunger; desire for cool air or to be fanned

- Coldness of breath; sweat, especially injured parts

Give *Carbo vegetabilis* 30C every fifteen to thirty minutes for three doses, less often as symptoms improve.

COMMONSENSE MEASURES

- Call for emergency help immediately.

- Do not move the person if he or she is seriously injured.

- If possible have the person lie on his or her back with legs slightly elevated.

- Loosen the clothing and warm the person with blankets, but avoid overheating.

- Offer reassurance and a drink of water to which a few drops of Rescue Remedy have been added, but only if the person is alert.

SEEK PROFESSIONAL HELP
- Immediately

SPLINTERS

Splinters are usually minor irritations and can be removed with a sterilized needle or tweezers. Bathe the area with *Hypericum* and *Calendula* tincture for pain and to prevent infection. Hypercal ointment may also be applied to soothe the spot. *Silica* may be given internally to aid the body in expelling splinters if there are many or they are difficult to remove. Also a few *Silica* pellets may be added to several ounces of water and the injured part soaked in the solution. Repeat two or three times per day to speed the expulsion of splinters. Note: *Silica* should not be used internally by anyone with a cardiac pacemaker or any surgically implanted artificial parts (such as an IUD or joint replacement) unless under the guidance of a qualified homeopath.

SILICA
Silica 6X or 6C may be given four times per day for up to ten days.

SPRAINS, STRAINS, AND SORE MUSCLES

A *sprain* is an injury around a joint causing the muscles, ligaments, or tendons to be stretched or torn, resulting in tenderness, pain, and swelling. The most commonly affected areas are ankles, wrists, knees, and fingers. A *strain* is a muscle injury that causes stretching or tearing of the muscle fibers, resulting in swelling and pain. Strains of the back muscles are most common, often resulting from lifting or twisting. Even when these injuries need medical care, homeopathy can effectively support the healing process. (See also "Back Injuries and Backache.")

The following remedies may be given every one to three hours, depending on the severity of symptoms, during the first day. Give as needed thereafter, up to four times per day, less often as symptoms improve.

ARNICA MONTANA

- Primary remedy for sprains and strains

- Sore, aching pain; prominent swelling and bruising

- For initial shock of the injury

Arnica is the premier remedy for any trauma or injury. It can greatly reduce pain, swelling, and bruising. After the initial shock either continue giving *Arnica* or change to one of the following remedies.

BRYONIA ALBA

- Swelling of joints

- Joint or muscle pains that may be especially sharp or stitching

- Worse from the slightest movement, even breathing

Bryonia is useful for sprains and strains in which even the slightest motion causes pain. Unlike for *Rhus toxicodendron,* the pain is not relieved by continued motion but is worsened.

RHUS TOXICODENDRON

- Sprained joints; swelling around joints

- Pulled muscles, torn ligaments, tendonitis

- Much pain with marked stiffness; restlessness

- Worse from first movements after rest, from cold

- Better from continued gentle motion, rubbing, firm pressure, and warmth

Rhus toxicodendron is a highly effective remedy for many strains and sprains and often follows *Arnica*. It is often called the rusty gate remedy, since it is used when pain and stiffness are worse during initial movement and are eased with continued gentle motion. *Rhus toxicodendron* will reduce pain and swelling, and help to heal the injury.

RUTA GRAVEOLENS

- Torn or overstretched ligaments and tendons

- Damage to cartilage

- Bruised bones close to the surface of the skin; shinsplints

Ruta may follow *Arnica* after the shock of the injury. It is best used when the initial swelling and pain have begun to subside. *Ruta* is especially valuable in wrist and ankle injuries and is also used for bruises to bone coverings (periosteum), such as around the shinbone.

STRONTIUM CARBONICUM

- Lingering pain after an ankle or wrist sprain

Strontium is useful in ankle or wrist injuries that have not healed well. If there is persistent or lingering pain after other remedies have been tried, *Strontium* may help. It is also a good remedy for repeated ankle or wrist injuries. Constitutional homeopathic treatment may be warranted if a person has this tendency. Give one dose of *Strontium* 6X or 6C three times per day for up to three weeks.

COMMONSENSE MEASURES

- Rest is essential for both the injured part and the person.

- Elevate the injured part and apply an ice pack during the first twenty-four to forty-eight hours to keep swelling down.

- Afterward a warm compress or a soak in a warm bath can relieve soreness, stiffness, and knotted muscles. To further ease the discomfort you may add to the bath 1 cup of Epsom salts or ½ cup each of baking soda and sea salt.

- Apply firm pressure with a bandage and keep it on during all other times.

- On unbroken skin you may use *Arnica* ointment or oil, or Traumed ointment. Massage it in three or four times per day while there is pain. Ease back into normal activity.

Reduce the risk of such injuries by stretching and doing warm-ups before vigorous exercise. Overzealous weekend athletes are especially vulnerable to sprains and strains. If you have a tendency to injure a certain part, massage it with *Arnica* oil and put on an elastic support *before* heading to the ball field, tennis court, or gym. And put some *Arnica* in your gym bag.

SEEK PROFESSIONAL HELP

- If pain persists or is severe

- If an injured joint looks distorted or unusually loose

- If the injured part is cold, blue, or numb

- If the injured part is impossible to move

PART 4

ACUTE AILMENTS AND THEIR TREATMENT

ALLERGIES AND HAY FEVER

Homeopathic medicines can be very effective in helping alleviate the acute symptoms of seasonal respiratory allergies. Allergies are viewed as a sign of a deeper underlying imbalance and, when symptoms are chronic or recur regularly, constitutional treatment is necessary to achieve deep and lasting results. The following remedies may be used for the short-term, seasonal treatment of hay fever.

ALLIUM CEPA
- Profuse, watery nasal discharge that feels like a running faucet

- Acrid and burning nasal discharge, often irritating the nose or upper lip

- Profuse tearing of eyes, usually bland (opposite *Euphrasia*)

- Eyes may be red and burning; desire to rub eyes

- Sneezing with rawness and tingling; frontal headache

- Worse from the smell of flowers, in the late afternoon or evening, from being in a warm room; better in the open air

AMBROSIA
- Hay fever from exposure to ragweed

- Intolerable itching of eyelids

- Tearing, burning eyes and watery nasal discharge

- May be asthmatic breathing, wheezing, or coughing

___

ARSENICUM ALBUM
- Burning tears and watery nasal discharge, often worse on the right side

- Nose may be completely stopped up even though it is dripping

- Difficult breathing during allergies; may be asthmatic

- Anxiety and restlessness

- Worse after midnight

- Person feels chilly and is better in a warm room

- Thirst for small sips

___

ARUNDO
- Marked itching on the roof of the mouth and inside nostrils (compare *Wyethia*)

- Runny nose with loss of smell and sneezing

- Increased salivation

___

DULCAMARA
- Hay fever at the end of summer or early fall

- During change in weather, especially from warm to cold

- Sinusitis with thick yellow mucus and facial pain

___

EUPHRASIA
- Profuse burning tears and bland nasal discharge (opposite *Allium cepa*)

- Eyes burn and are very sensitive to light; much blinking

- Eyes and cheeks reddened from acrid tears

- Eye symptoms worse in open air

- Nasal discharge worse when lying down and at night

NATRUM MURIATICUM

- Symptoms develop after grief, loss, or suppression of emotions

- Frequent sneezing; watery discharge from eyes and nose, like egg whites

- In later stages nasal mucus becomes thick and white

- Sense of smell and taste lost

- Symptoms worse in the morning; coughing up of mucus

- Headache from exposure to sun

NUX VOMICA

- Nasal discharge flows during the day and is congested at night

- Sneezing and runny nose worse in the morning on waking or rising

- Markedly irritable temperament, cross and impatient

- Itchiness inside ears

- Eyes sensitive to light

- Worse indoors; better in open air

PULSATILLA

- Nasal discharge flows during the day and is congested at night

- Congestion worse during warm weather and in a warm room; better in a cool environment or open air

- Marked sneezing and itchy, red eyes

- Thirstlessness, even with a dry mouth

- Person may be mild, tearful, and impressionable; desiring attention and sympathy

SABADILLA

- Violent sneezing is the primary complaint

- Sneezing that comes on in fits: many sneezes in a row

- Itching and tingling in nose

- Profuse thin nasal discharge

- Sneezing is worse in cold air and from odors and perfumes

WYETHIA

- Marked itching in nose, throat, and roof of the mouth (compare *Arundo*)

- Person must "cluck" with the back of the tongue to soothe itching

- Irritation in the throat; constant clearing of the throat; throat feels swollen

- Sneezing and dry cough

COMMONSENSE MEASURES

- To help strengthen your resistance to pollens, eat a small amount of raw honey each day. Honey gathered from your local area can provide a natural means of enhancing immunity over time. Other helpful measures for acute allergy symptoms include freeze-dried stinging nettle (*Urtica dioica*) taken in capsule form three times daily; flaxseed oil, 1 teaspoon taken twice daily; vitamin C with bioflavonoids, 500 mg four times per day; and nasal douching with a saltwater solution. A neti pot, used in Ayurvedic medicine from India, is a convenient device for nasal douching.

- If you are blowing your nose frequently, prevent dryness and irritation by applying *Calendula* cream or another plant-based healing salve.

- Be extremely cautious of conventional allergy treatments. Many of them can further damage immunity with suppressive therapies. Consult a homeopath or other natural health care provider for further treatment of chronic or recurrent allergies.

APPENDICITIS (SEE ALSO "DIGESTIVE PROBLEMS: ABDOMINAL PAIN")

Marked pain in the lower right abdomen that is accompanied by nausea and vomiting may indicate appendicitis. Additional signs that may confirm it are

- Guarding—stiffening of the abdominal muscles when one is approached

- Rebound tenderness: The area is not painful when pressed, but significant pain is felt when pressure is released

Homeopathic treatment has been known to arrest the progress of appendicitis in some cases. However, always seek medical care if you suspect this condition. Give one of the following remedies en route to the doctor or emergency room. A 30C potency is preferred, given at ten- to thirty-minute intervals depending on the severity of symptoms. Repeat the dose at least until medical help arrives, then continue when possible.

ACONITE

- Sudden onset of abdominal pains following exposure to cold weather

- Anxiety, fear, and restlessness

- Worse from sneezing or jarring; pains may extend to chest or shoulder

BELLADONNA

- Sharp and severe abdominal pains or cramps that come and go suddenly

- Markedly worse from motion and jarring; worse lying on the painful side

- Better from lying on abdomen or applying steady pressure

BRYONIA ALBA

- Primary remedy for appendicitis

- Pain from the slightest motion; must lie completely still

- Pain sharp, sore, or stitching

- Worse from any motion, coughing, deep breathing

- Better from lying on the painful side

SEEK PROFESSIONAL HELP

- Immediately if you suspect appendicitis

ATHLETE'S FOOT

Athlete's foot is a chronic or recurrent skin condition for some people. In such cases constitutional homeopathic care is advisable. To prevent recurrence keep the feet clean, dry them carefully after washing, and expose them to air and sunshine as often as possible. Swab affected areas with distilled white vinegar several times a day in stubborn cases. Dust them with *Calendula* baby powder to absorb perspiration and use *Calendula* ointment on any cracked or painful areas. *Thuja* ointment may also be applied during flare-ups. Avoid the use of antifungal powders, creams, and foot antiperspirants. These are suppressive and can lead to other health problems.

GRAPHITES

- Moist, oozing eruptions and thick crusts

- Toenails thickened, distorted, and/or crumbly

SULPHUR

- Extreme itchiness with marked burning

- In warm-blooded people who have *Sulphur* characteristics

SEEK PROFESSIONAL HELP

- If there is much pain or inflammation

CANKER SORES/COLD SORES

The following remedies are often effective in treating sores in the mouth. Canker sores, cold sores (fever blisters), and mouth ulcers typically appear when a person is under stress, run down, or has a cold or fever. Cold sores are considered manifestations of the herpes simplex virus, Type I. The following remedies can be quite helpful for an outbreak of most types of mouth sores, although a recurrent problem indicates the need for constitutional treatment.

Select a remedy and give one dose of 12C or 30C, three to four times per day for three days, less often as symptoms improve.

ARSENICUM ALBUM

- Markedly burning ulcers or sores relieved by heat or warm drinks
- Vesicles (small blisters) that break open, leaving ulcerated spots
- Pain worse at night

BORAX

- A primary remedy for sores in the mouth
- Ulcers or canker sores in the mouth or on the tongue
- Ulcers that feel hot or bleed
- Sores that cause much pain when eating or sucking

MERCURIUS

- Excessive salivation with mouth sores; drooling on pillow
- Offensive breath

NATRUM MURIATICUM

- A primary remedy for sores of the mouth
- Herpes eruptions on lips, translucent or like little pearls
- Dry lips; often cracked in the corners or in the center of lower lip
- Dry mouth with much thirst; patchy eruptions inside mouth; patchy tongue
- Outbreak after an emotional upset or exposure to sun

RHUS TOXICODENDRON

- Like *Natrum mur*, herpetic eruptions and dry cracking in corners of lips

- Red, itching, burning eruptions

- Much restlessness and difficulty sleeping

- From exposure to damp or cold weather

SEPIA

- Cold sores; especially of the lower lip, which is often cracked or chapped

- Eruptions occur during menstruation or ovulation

SULPHUR

- Mouth ulcers that burn; small blisters in patches

- Offensive breath

- If *Mercurius* and other remedies have not helped

- Worse at night; from heat of bed

COMMONSENSE MEASURES

- Gargle with either *Calendula* or *Hydrastis* (goldenseal) tincture diluted with water: add 1 dropperful to 4 ounces of warm water.

- Ipsab herbal mouth and gum treatment, a solution containing prickly ash bark, can be very soothing and healing. Apply the concentrate directly with a cotton swab three or four times per day or as needed.

- Vitamin C with bioflavonoids may be taken, 2000 mg daily for up to five days.

- Avoidance of chocolate, nuts, seeds, and a variety of grains is helpful for some people with cold sores.

- The amino acid *lysine* is well known to be a beneficial supplement for people with herpes.

SEEK PROFESSIONAL HELP

- If the condition recurs with regularity

- If symptoms are severe or the preceding measures are not helping

COLDS, COUGHS, AND BRONCHITIS

Many common colds and coughs can occur along with other complaints, such as sore throat, fever, flu symptoms, or sinus infection.
Treatment of each condition can be found in its own section of this
book. If you have two or more ailments, for instance, a cold with a
sore throat, you should consult both the cold section and the sore
throat section to make the most accurate selection of remedy. There
are many, many remedies for colds, coughs, and bronchitis. Only the
most commonly used remedies appear here.

During the onset of any cold, cough, or bronchitis symptoms,
Aconite, Belladonna, and *Ferrum phosphoricum* should be considered. If
none of these is indicated, proceed to other remedy options for those
conditions. When the onset is sudden and strong, such as in cases
that require *Aconite* or *Belladonna,* the dose should be repeated more
frequently: every fifteen minutes to one hour depending on severity.
Generally, in cases where symptoms are less forceful or appear more
gradually, give one dose every three or four hours.

For the initial onset of symptoms of colds, coughs, or bronchitis,
consider these three remedies:

ACONITE

- During the first twenty-four hours of symptoms

- Sudden and forceful onset of symptoms after exposure to dry,
  cold, or windy weather

- Marked restlessness, anxiety, and fear

- High fever

- A dry cough may be present, worse at night

BELLADONNA

- During the first twenty-four hours of symptoms

- Sudden and forceful onset with high fever

- Face is dry and flushed red; head is hot; hands and feet are cool

- Eyes may be red or glazed and are sensitive to light

- Sore throat may be present

FERRUM PHOSPHORICUM

- Early stages of a cold or cough; the first twenty-four to forty-eight hours

- No strongly distinguishing symptoms

- Onset is not sudden or intense, as with *Aconite* or *Belladonna*

- Fever and flushed cheeks

- Hoarseness and dry cough may be present

COLDS

The common cold is aptly named, because almost everyone gets a cold from time to time. It is the habit of our modern times to take a pill for every ill. But it is not necessary to take a remedy every time a sniffle comes on. As long as our bodies are given the chance to clean house without suppressing nasal discharges or fever, many minor cases can be overcome with commonsense support. However, if illness comes on forcefully, the healing process is slow, or suffering is great, a homeopathic remedy can bring relief and rapid healing.

ALLIUM CEPA

- Profuse, watery nasal discharge; feels like a running faucet

- Nasal discharge is acrid and burning, often irritating the nose or upper lip

- Profuse tearing of eyes, usually bland (opposite *Euphrasia*)

- Eyes may be red and burning; desire to rub eyes

- Sneezing with rawness and tingling; tickling in larynx; frontal headache

- Worse from being in a warm room; better in open air

ARSENICUM ALBUM

- Burning, irritating, watery nasal discharge, often worse on the right side

- Nose may feel completely stopped up, even though it is dripping

- Anxiety and restlessness; fear of being alone

- Chilly and sensitive to drafts; better in a warm room

- Thirst for small sips taken frequently

- Symptoms may be worse after midnight

DULCAMARA

- Symptoms that appear after exposure to cold, wet weather

- From becoming chilled or wet after being very warm

- Colds during transition from late summer to fall; warm days, cold nights

EUPHRASIA

- Profuse burning tears and bland nasal discharge (opposite *Allium cepa*)

- Eyes burn and are very sensitive to light; much blinking

- Acrid tears redden eyes and cheeks

- Eye symptoms worse in open air

- Nasal discharge and sneezing worse when lying down and at night

- Hoarseness; cough in daytime only, better lying down and at night

___

GELSEMIUM

- Gradual onset of symptoms; often during warm, humid weather

- Great weakness, dullness; heavy feeling and dizziness

- Sneezing and watery nasal discharge

- Low-grade fever; body aches; chills running up and down back

- Face may be dusky red; drooping eyelids

- Desire to lie still and be left alone

___

HEPAR SULPHURIS

- Sneezing from the least draft of cold air

- Extreme sensitivity to touch, pain, anything cold

- Thick, yellow nasal discharge

- Nose feels very sore

- Irritability

___

KALI BICHROMICUM

- Thick nasal discharge that is stringy, ropy, or gluey, like rubber cement

- Postnasal drip adheres to back of throat or nose, difficult to expel

- Worse in the cold or open air

NUX VOMICA
- Symptoms often develop after overindulgence in food, alcohol, or drugs

- Very chilly, must stay bundled up; slight movement brings on chills

- Marked irritability; short-tempered or bossy

- Watery nasal discharge in the daytime, blocked nose at night

PULSATILLA
- Thick, bland, creamy nasal discharge; usually yellow or greenish

- Nasal congestion worse in a stuffy, warm room; better in open air

- Moody, easily brought to tears; craving company and sympathy

- Usually thirstless

COUGHS
Coughs may occur along with a cold or fever and can range from mild nuisances to painful, debilitating, and quite serious chest conditions. Only coughs and bronchitis will be covered here. For croup, consult Part 5. If coughs are a recurrent problem, constitutional treatment should be sought. For the earlier stages of cough, see the indications of *Aconite*, *Belladonna*, and *Ferrum phos* at the beginning of "Colds, Coughs, and Bronchitis."

ANTIMONIUM TARTARICUM
- Weakness and debility with deep, wet, rattling cough

- Winter coughs in elderly people

- (See "Bronchitis")

BRYONIA ALBA

- Dry cough after a cold has moved down into the chest

- Hard, painful cough; must hold chest while coughing

- Cough and pain worse from any motion, from breathing deeply

- Pain through head and chest with every cough

- Desire to remain still

- Thirst for cold drinks

- Cough aggravated by eating and in a warm room; better in open air

- Nausea or vomiting may be present

DROSERA

- Dry, barking cough

- Tickling in throat excites cough

- Bouts of choking cough may end in retching or vomiting

- (See "Croup")

DULCAMARA

- (See "Bronchitis")

HEPAR SULPHURIS

- "Ripe" colds and coughs with thick yellow mucus

- Barking, croupy cough

- Cough from exposure to cold
- (See "Croup" or "Bronchitis")

___

KALI BICHROMICUM
- More typically for later stages of a cough
- Cough that produces thick yellow or greenish mucus
- Mucus from chest or nose is tough, ropy, stringy, or gluey
- Tickling in back of throat excites cough; hoarseness

___

PHOSPHORUS
- Cough that begins with a cold and descends into chest
- Dry, hard cough; worse from talking, laughing, or going from a warm room into cool air
- Cough from tickling behind sternum
- Cough worse when lying, especially on the left side
- Craving for iced or cold drinks, though chilly
- Nosebleed or blood-tinged nasal mucus
- Fear of the dark, desire for company

___

PULSATILLA
- Dry cough during the day, productive wet cough at night and in the morning
- Coughing worse in a warm room; better in open air and with gentle walking
- Yellow or greenish mucus from cough
- Cough worse lying; better from sitting up or lying with head propped up

- Person may be mild and affectionate; craves reassurance and company, weeps easily

RHUS TOXICODENDRON
- Symptoms appear after getting wet or chilled

- Marked restlessness

- Cough, hoarseness, and sore throat; better from warm drinks

- Chills and cough at night; tossing and turning, cannot settle down

RUMEX
- Cough from tickling in throat pit, touching throat aggravates cough

- Markedly worse from inhaling cold air, which triggers cough

- Person covers mouth with hand or blanket to breathe in warmer air

- Cough worse on waking in the morning or at 11:00 P.M.

- (See "Croup")

SPONGIA TOSTA
- Primary remedy for dry and croupy coughs

- Dry cough: like a seal's bark or a saw going through wood

- Cough better from eating or drinking, especially warm drinks

- (See "Croup")

BRONCHITIS
Bronchitis can occur when a cold or cough settles in the chest. There may be difficult or noisy breathing, wheezing, or rattling. Some

people have a tendency to get bronchitis seasonally or repeatedly. To uproot this problem constitutional treatment is recommended. Select one of the following remedies for relief of acute bronchitis.

For the earliest stages of bronchitis, see the indications of *Aconite*, *Belladonna*, and *Ferrum phos* at the beginning of "Colds, Coughs, and Bronchitis."

ANTIMONIUM TARTARICUM
- Weakness and debility in advanced coughs and bronchitis
- Marked drowsiness during bronchitis
- Rattling mucus; deep, wet cough but very little mucus is brought up
- Sweaty and pale face; blueness may be present around lips
- Irritability, aversion to being touched

BRYONIA ALBA
- (See "Coughs")

DULCAMARA
- Bronchitis after exposure to cold, wet weather
- Bronchitis after getting chilled or wet after being very warm, or during transition from late summer to fall
- Loose, wet cough that produces much mucus; worse from exertion
- Herpes eruptions on lips may be present

HEPAR SULPHURIS
- Marked chilliness; intolerance of becoming cold; desire for warm drinks

- Extreme oversensitivity: to pain, touch, drafts, or anything cold

- Splinterlike pains may be present in throat, chest, or ears

- Anxiety, irritability, critical disposition

- Night sweats

- (See "Croup")

IPECACUANHA

- Rapidly developing bronchitis with wheezing or asthmatic breathing

- Nausea, retching, or vomiting during cough

- Rattling, wet cough; worse in warm, humid weather

- Weakness and difficulty raising mucus

- Spasmodic, choking cough

- Nosebleed during cough

- (See "Croup")

KALI CARBONICUM

- Cough or wheezing worse between 2:00 and 4:00 A.M.

- Chilly, sensitive to drafts and cold air

- Tickling sensation in throat on first lying down at night

- Symptoms worse lying flat; better from sitting up or bending forward (compare *Pulsatilla*)

PHOSPHORUS

- Wheezing or coughing worse from talking, laughing, or going from a warm room into cool air

- Chest feels tight or constricted

- Craving for iced or cold drinks, though chilly

- Nosebleed or blood-tinged nasal mucus

- Anxiety and fear of the dark; desire for company

PULSATILLA

- Difficult breathing and coughing worse at night in bed and in the morning

- Symptoms worse lying flat; better lying propped up with pillows or sitting up (compare *Kali carb*)

- Symptoms worse from emotions, in a warm room; better in open air

- Yellow or greenish mucus with cough

- Person may be mild, affectionate, and weepy, craving reassurance and company

- Little or no thirst, even with fever; dry lips

COMMONSENSE MEASURES

In addition to a homeopathic remedy, some simple home care measures may prevent the illness from progressing further and lessen its severity or duration:

- Allow for adequate rest, the closer to onset the better. Don't wait for symptoms to knock you over before giving in to rest. Minimize external stressors as much as possible.

- At the earliest sign of illness, squeeze the juice of one lemon into a tall glass of hot water. Add a small pinch of cayenne pepper and stir. Drink at bedtime and again on waking in the morning, taking no food within an hour. This helps to cleanse and prevent backup of mucus in the body.

- Moderate the diet. Take simple, smaller, easy-to-digest meals that do not overtax the system. Reduce or eliminate sugar, caffeine, and fatty foods. Take extra clear fluids, preferably warm, noncaffeinated teas. Any fruit juices should be diluted 50 percent with warm water. Only *fresh-squeezed* orange juice contains enough vitamin C to be of benefit.

- Steam inhalation can be very soothing to the nose, throat, and chest and will help loosen congestion. Running a hot shower in a closed bathroom is a convenient way to create steam. Also excellent is a chamomile steam inhalation: Put a small handful of loose chamomile flowers in the bottom of a large mixing bowl. Pour boiling water over the flowers to fill the bowl halfway. Sit with your face above the bowl, and drape a large towel over your head and the bowl to create a tent. Inhale slowly and deeply for ten or fifteen minutes. Use caution near hot water. Repeat twice per day or as needed.

- Extra vitamin C can be beneficial: 500 mg four times per day for up to one week.

- Echinacea: 20 to 30 drops in tea or water twice per day for up to one week during early stages of illness.

- For early stages of coughs, colds, and sore throats, zinc lozenges are often very beneficial.

SEEK PROFESSIONAL HELP

- If the condition worsens or symptoms are prolonged or severe

- If the preceding measures do not help

DIGESTIVE PROBLEMS

Digestive problems encompass a wide variety of ailments: abdominal pain, constipation, diarrhea, gas, indigestion, nausea, and vomiting. Often one condition occurs with another, such as indigestion with constipation. When this is the case, cross-reference the symptoms in the appropriate sections before choosing a remedy.

The following remedies can bring relief for a wide range of acute digestive complaints. Chronic problems may require lifestyle and dietary changes as well as constitutional treatment. Conditions that warrant medical attention are listed at the end of each section.

ABDOMINAL PAIN

Abdominal pain can be caused by a variety of factors including infections; inflammation of the stomach, bowels, intestines, or appendix; gallstones; kidney stones; or menstrual problems. Symptoms such as gas or indigestion may also contribute to abdominal pain. Even when the exact diagnosis is not known, the symptom picture can effectively indicate which homeopathic remedy will give relief.

For conditions that warrant prompt medical attention, a remedy can be given en route to the doctor or emergency room. (See also "Appendicitis.")

ACONITE

- Sudden onset of abdominal pains following exposure to cold weather

- After a fright or shock

- Anxiety, fear, and restlessness

- Worse from sneezing or jarring; may extend to chest or shoulder

ARSENICUM ALBUM

- Burning abdominal pain; may be accompanied by diarrhea and/or vomiting

- Worse after midnight; from cold weather and cold food

- Anxiety and restlessness; weakness and marked chilliness

- Better from warmth and drinking milk

BELLADONNA

- Sharp and severe abdominal pains or cramps that come and go suddenly

- Worse from motion and jarring, and lying on the painful side

- Better from lying on abdomen or applying steady pressure

BRYONIA ALBA

- Primary remedy for appendicitis and many abdominal conditions

- Pain from the slightest motion; must lie completely still

- Pains sharp, sore, or stitching

- Worse from any motion, coughing, deep breathing

- Better from lying on the painful side

CHAMOMILLA

- Intense anger or irritability from pain; nothing pleases

- Arching the back during pain; painful cramping

- Greenish diarrhea that looks like chopped spinach

- Worse at night, from eating, from coffee, after a fit of anger

- Better from warmth

CHELIDONIUM MAJUS

- Pain in the region of the gallbladder

- Deep, stitching pains in the upper right portion of abdomen; constriction across abdomen, as from a string

- Pains that radiate to right shoulder or shoulder blade

- Pain comes on after eating fats; worse from pressure

- Better from warm milk, warm food or drinks

_____

COLOCYNTHIS

- Severe constricting or cramping pains; better from bending double

- Pains that follow anger or indignation; from taking offense

- Twisting and writhing with pain; relieved by writhing or rolling about

- Constipation, diarrhea, or nausea may accompany pain

- Better from applying warmth, hard pressure, walking bent over, motion

_____

LYCOPODIUM

- Pain on the right side of abdomen

- Bloating, distension, and loud rumbling

- Aggravated by onions, cabbage, oysters, wheat

- Worse between 4:00 and 8:00 P.M. or in the morning, when lying on the right side

- Better from warm drinks, loosening clothing, and temporarily from belching or passing gas

_____

MAGNESIA PHOSPHORICA

- Cramping and constricting pains similar to *Colocynthis*

- Better from application of strong heat, hot drinks, firm pressure, bending double

NUX VOMICA

- Painful spasms and cramping, often with nausea

- Frequent but ineffectual urge to move bowels, even with loose stool

- Irritability and oversensitivity to all stimuli

- Worse from cold, pressure, jarring, spicy foods, alcohol, and coffee

- Better from warmth and after bowel movements

SEEK PROFESSIONAL HELP

- Abdominal pain that is caused by problems such as kidney stones, gallstones, hepatitis, or appendicitis requires prompt professional care even if a remedy is helping. If the cause of acute pain is not known, use common sense and seek medical advice when pain is severe or does not improve within a reasonable time.

CONSTIPATION

Constipation can often be prevented with adequate fluids and fiber in the diet, and through exercise and stress management. Anxiety, worries, and tension, as well as traveling away from home often adversely affect regular elimination. Prune juice is a time-honored aid for relief of occasional constipation; try drinking it hot for the best effect. Avoid laxatives, which are habit forming and ultimately worsen the condition. If constipation is a recurrent problem, seek constitutional homeopathic care. For relief of acute symptoms, the following remedies will stimulate the body's ability to restore balance.

ALUMINA

- No urge to move bowels

- Stools may be hard, knotty, and dry

- Stools also may be soft, quite sticky, and difficult to wipe clean

- Hard to expel even when stool is soft

- Craving for dry, starchy foods, such as rice or potatoes, yet made worse by them

- Sedentary habits or while traveling

- Eating foods prepared with aluminum cookware

BRYONIA ALBA

- Large stools that are hard, dry, and difficult to expel

- Irritable, grumpy, wants to be left alone

- Dryness of both rectum and mouth; much thirst for cold drinks

- Any motion aggravates abdominal discomfort; desire to remain still

CALCAREA CARBONICA

- No urge to move bowels, can go on for days

- Person feels comfortable when constipated

- Craving for eggs, starches, cold drinks

- Milk intolerance, which can cause constipation or other complaints

- Lethargy, poor stamina; phlegmatic

NUX VOMICA

- Constant or frequent urge to move bowels

- Ineffectual urging, produces only a small amount, even a soft stool

- "Never quite finished" feeling after bowel movements

- Best remedy for people with recent history of laxative use

- Hard, painful stools; while traveling

- Irritability and oversensitivity to cold and all stimuli

SEPIA

- Often a remedy for women during hormonal changes: menstruation, menopause, pregnancy, or postpartum

- Ineffectual urging, similar to *Nux vomica;* or no urging

- Sensation of a ball in rectum

- Person may be overly critical or indifferent to loved ones

- Better from vigorous exercise, dancing, or when busy

SILICA

- "Bashful" stool, one that is partially expelled and then slips back inside rectum

- Great difficulty and straining to pass even a soft stool

- Chilly and sensitive to cold; tendency to be intolerant to milk

- Easy perspiration of head, hands, and feet

- Person may be timid, delicate, and/or overly conscientious about details

COMMONSENSE MEASURES

- Overall moderation in diet is very helpful.

- Avoid the foods (or quantities of foods) that are known to result in digestive problems.

- Chew thoroughly before swallowing food. Slowing down can make a big difference.

- Promptly heed the urge to empty the bowels.

- Apply a hot water bottle to the abdomen if it gives relief.

- Sipping ginger tea or chamomile tea may be helpful in many digestive complaints. Brew chamomile tea for one minute only, and strain it before drinking.

SEEK PROFESSIONAL HELP

- If symptoms are recurrent or persistent

- If symptoms are severe or are not relieved within a reasonable time by the preceding measures

- If the person has a history of serious abdominal or digestive illness

DIARRHEA

Acute diarrhea can occur after eating foods that are not well tolerated, including contaminated food, and during influenza, or after an emotional upset. Persistent diarrhea can cause dehydration and lead to other health problems. Therefore, fluid intake should be encouraged as part of the treatment and recovery process. Diarrhea that is recurrent or chronic should be addressed by a professional homeopath and may also need medical evaluation. See also "Food Poisoning" or "Influenza."

ACONITE

- Sudden onset after a fright or exposure to cold weather

- Anxiety, restlessness, and fear

ALOE

- Much gas expelled with stool

- Involuntary stools or insecure feeling in rectum (must hold it in)

- Gurgling and rumbling before bowel movements

ARGENTUM NITRICUM

- Nervousness, anticipatory anxiety; stage fright

- Often accompanied by flatulence

- Worse after consuming sugar

ARSENICUM ALBUM

- Great weakness and exhaustion

- Food poisoning, stomach flu, or travelers' diarrhea

- Diarrhea with vomiting, may occur simultaneously

- Cramping and burning pain; burning in anus from irritating stool

- From eating fruit

- Chilly, anxious, and restless

CHAMOMILLA

- Diarrhea with cramping pains

- Stool often greenish, resembling chopped spinach or grass

- Intense irritability; may come on after a fit of anger

IPECACUANHA

- Diarrhea accompanied by marked and persistent nausea not relieved by vomiting

- Tongue pink and clean despite stomach upset

NUX VOMICA

- Constant urge to move bowels but can pass only small amounts

- After overeating, alcohol, tobacco, coffee, or drugs

- Marked irritability or impatience

- Oversensitivity to cold and all stimuli

PHOSPHORUS

- From slight aberrations in the diet

- Watery, painless stool

- Rectum feels loose or open

- Thirsty for cold water or juice

PODOPHYLLUM

- Profuse, explosive, forcefully ejected stool

- Much rumbling and gurgling before stool

- Stool may be watery or mucusy, and very offensive smelling

- Often occurs in summer

SULPHUR

- Urgent diarrhea first thing in the morning, or around 5:00 or 6:00 A.M.

- Markedly offensive smelling stool, often like rotten eggs

- Anus may be red, itching, or burning

- Worse from sour foods, sweets, milk, and beer

VERATRUM ALBUM

- Diarrhea with vomiting, often occurring simultaneously

- Profuse, odorless, watery stool

- Trembling, cold sweat, pale face

- Very chilly, weak, and exhausted

GAS

Excess gas forming in the stomach and intestines occurs when the digestive process is out of balance. Eating more slowly and chewing thoroughly helps to break down food better, making gas less likely. A variety of stresses can also play a role in digestive problems. Whatever the cause, a homeopathic remedy can help the body restore balance.

ARGENTUM NITRICUM
- Much loud and intense flatulence and belching

- After eating sweets

- Worse from anxiety

CARBO VEGETABILIS
- Tremendous bloating from any kind of food, about half an hour after eating

- Frequent belching, which helps alleviate the discomfort

- Flatulence may be worse at night and when lying down

- Marked craving for fresh air or being fanned

CHINA
- Trapped abdominal gas that won't easily move up or down

- Rumbling and distension; cramping

- Passing gas and belching do not relieve discomfort

- Aggravated by fruit, milk, fat, and beer

LYCOPODIUM

- Bloating and distension, even from eating a small amount of food

- Loud rumbling

- Discomfort relieved temporarily by belching and passing gas

- Aggravated by onions, cabbage, oysters, wheat

- Symptoms may be worse between 4:00 and 8:00 P.M., or in the morning on rising

INDIGESTION

Indigestion is a term used to describe a variety of acute abdominal discomforts that develop after eating. Simply slowing down or eating less at mealtimes can help prevent symptoms such as heartburn, queasiness, belching, and gas. Other factors that can contribute to indigestion include poor diet and mental or emotional stress. The following remedies will help alleviate occasional digestive upset.

ARSENICUM ALBUM

- Marked burning in esophagus and stomach

- Desire for frequent small sips of water

- Worse from cold food and drinks

- Better from warm drinks or milk

BRYONIA ALBA

- Heaviness, like a stone, in stomach after eating

- Bitter belching

- Worse from the least movement

- Great thirst for cold drinks

- May be accompanied by constipation

CARBO VEGETABILIS

- Tremendous bloating with indigestion about half an hour after eating

- Frequent belching, which helps alleviate discomfort

- Heartburn and gas

- Marked craving for fresh air or being fanned

CHAMOMILLA

- Indigestion following a fit of anger or irritability

- Distended abdomen and painful cramping

- Bitter taste in mouth

- May be accompanied by greenish diarrhea

NUX VOMICA

- Indigestion after overindulgence in food, alcohol, coffee, or tobacco

- Cramping, spasms, or sharp pains; heartburn, belching with bitter reflux; bloating

- Frequent but ineffective urging to belch or move bowels

- Better from warmth or warm drinks

PULSATILLA

- Indigestion from fats and rich foods, ice cream, pork

- Bloating and nausea; no thirst

- Feeling peevish, weepy, or whiny; desiring sympathy

NAUSEA AND VOMITING

Acute nausea and vomiting often occur after eating and drinking too much, eating contaminated food, or with influenza. (See also "Food Poisoning," "Influenza," "Motion Sickness.")

ANTIMONIUM CRUDUM

- Vomiting from overeating, especially rich or indigestible foods

- Vomiting soon after eating or drinking

- Tongue coated white

- Irritability; does not want to be looked at

ARSENICUM ALBUM

- Food poisoning or stomach flu

- Great weakness and exhaustion

- Vomiting and diarrhea may occur simultaneously

- Burning in esophagus and stomach, relieved by heat or warm drinks

- Desire for small sips of water, but may be vomited shortly after

- Anxiety and restlessness; much fear with vomiting; fear of being alone

BRYONIA ALBA

- Slow onset of flu with body aches, headache

- All symptoms made worse by any motion; must lie very still

- Better from cold drinks and being left alone

CARBO VEGETABILIS

- Severe nausea with marked coldness, pallor, and great weakness

- Constant desire to belch, which gives some relief

- Strong desire for cool, open air or being fanned

IPECACUANHA

- Persistent and severe nausea not relieved by vomiting

- Tongue pink and clean despite stomach upset

- Nausea and vomiting associated with coughs or bronchitis

- Offensive breath

NUX VOMICA

- Painful vomiting and retching; frequent ineffectual attempts to vomit

- From overindulgence in food, alcohol, or drugs

- Constipation and cramping

- Chilly, irritable, and oversensitive to all stimuli

PHOSPHORUS

- Burning in stomach

- Thirst for cool drinks but vomits as soon as liquid becomes warm in stomach

- Worse from warm food and drinks, smoke, odors

- Better from lying on the right side, sleep, temporarily from cold drinks

- Serious conditions with vomiting of blood

VERATRUM ALBUM

- Severe vomiting with diarrhea, often occurring simultaneously

- Projectile vomiting

- Chilliness, trembling, cold sweat on forehead, pallor

- Great weakness or collapse

EARACHE

Because earache is a far more common problem among children, the remedies and their indications can be found in Part 5. These remedies are perfectly serviceable for people of all ages.

EMOTIONAL CONDITIONS

Homeopathy is capable of stimulating profound emotional healing and has indeed helped many people with a wide variety of emotional difficulties. When prolonged or chronic, deeper emotional conditions are best addressed through constitutional treatment with a skilled homeopath. Often a trained and objective ear must listen at some length to a person's story in order for the most suitable remedy to be found. However, there are some acute emotional conditions that may be treated at home. The following is a small sampling of remedies that may be used, when indicated, on a short-term basis. If a remedy is well matched to a person's condition, give one dose of 30C from one to three times per day for up to one week, and review the section "Potency and Dosage Guidelines." If emotional difficulties are longstanding or if recent ones persist after one week, consider seeking out a qualified homeopath for help.

ANGER

NUX VOMICA

Nux vomica is a remedy for people who are highly ambitious, competitive, and driven to achieve. These Type A personalities are irritable, restless, impatient, and oftentimes have a tendency toward outbursts of anger and starting arguments. They can be quite bossy and intolerant of contradiction, and demand that others meet their high standards. Such people often crave stimulants (coffee, tobacco, alcohol) but are oversensitive to all kinds of stimuli: light, noise, odors—everything makes too strong an impression. With nerves on edge, they can easily snap at those around them or completely lose their temper. Their short fuses can make them likely perpetrators of road rage and even acts of violence.

STAPHYSAGRIA

A person who needs *Staphysagria* has deep anger that is strongly suppressed. Though the anger may be intensely felt, it is rarely expressed. In some instances, the suppression is so strong that he or she may be unaware of these feelings. Often such a person is the emotional doormat in the workplace or family situation and has covered this anger with a sweetness or mildness. Victims of rape, beatings, or emotional abuse often need this remedy, as do those living under severe domination (such as from a spouse, parent, boss, government) where the expression of anger is not tolerated. Whether or not such obviously harsh conditions are present, sexual shame is common, as is a general feeling of violation, humiliation, or victimization. Anger will occasionally be shown in the form of the person throwing things or slamming doors.

FEAR AND ANXIETY

ACONITE

Aconite is often needed after someone suffers a shock or a fright. After experiencing a natural disaster or witnessing a terrible accident, a person is beset by anxiety, panic episodes, or great terror. There is tremendous fear of death, and a certainty that death is imminent, even predicting the hour of death. After a shocking event, the person may wake during the night with fright. *Aconite* proved very helpful to people during the hours, days, and weeks following the attacks on the

World Trade Center. This remedy is also useful for children or adults who are terrified of visiting the doctor or dentist, displaying great anxiety, restlessness, and fear.

ARGENTUM NITRICUM

Argentum Nitricum is indicated by great nervousness and anxiety, with much apprehension about an upcoming event. This remedy is helpful when a person has performance anxiety (stage fright) or exam fears, dread of crossing a bridge, entering a tunnel or other closed-in place, fear of heights, or that a building will fall or collapse on him or her. A feeling of time pressure, as if anticipating something terrible, is common. The person tends to become hurried with anxiety and finds himself or herself walking faster and faster. Craving for sweets is strong, with diarrhea, flatulence, or belching often accompanying the nervousness.

ARSENICUM ALBUM

Arsenicum is for fear and anxiety in people who are tense, worried, and feel a strong need to control their environment. They tend to be obsessively neat, often dress immaculately, like their surroundings very orderly and clean, and are fearful about germs and contamination. Fears of death and disease are strong, and can become exacerbated especially when world events are focused on the threat of terrorism or epidemic diseases. Their anxiety about health can cause them to exaggerate minor symptoms and imagine they have an incurable disease. They dread being left alone and have a constant desire for company, with great dependency on others for a feeling of safety and security. Often tremendous restlessness is seen during bouts of anxiety. Anguishing fears can drive the person out of bed at night, causing him or her to pace or wander anxiously from room to room.

GELSEMIUM

People who need *Gelsemium* often feel a sinking lack of courage when facing an ordeal such as public speaking, an exam, performance, going to the doctor's office, or even childbirth. They are terror-stricken at the thought of the upcoming event. They tend to tremble, feel great mental and bodily weakness, dizziness, heaviness of the limbs, and want to withdraw from the ordeal. Desire for frequent urination is common.

LYCOPODIUM

Lycopodium is for people who have a marked lack of self-confidence, fear of failure, and a dread of undertaking anything new. They may be actually quite capable of meeting an upcoming challenge, but feel helpless because of low self-esteem. Exam fears and performance anxiety are common. They are extremely concerned about image and how people will perceive them, and worry that they will make complete fools of themselves. Those who need *Lycopodium* are attracted to people and places of power and may choose professions such as politics, law, or high-profile business, but they tend to avoid responsibility and commitment in their personal lives. They are usually agreeable at work but bossy at home. Some people who need *Lycopodium* project overconfidence and egotism, inflating themselves to compensate for low self-esteem. The abdomen also tends to be inflated, with gas and bloating being common ailments in those needing this remedy.

PHOSPHORUS

Phosphorus is a remedy for people who are highly sensitive to their surroundings and other people. They are receptive, impressionable, and suggestible, often with a lacking sense of boundaries, and are therefore easily beset by a variety of fears and anxieties. Common are fears of thunderstorms, darkness, being alone, imaginary things, ghosts or the supernatural, natural disaster, disease, and the health of loved ones. Often there is a pervasive, anxious feeling of foreboding—that something bad will happen. They are usually lively, open, and amiable, tend to have many friends, and are very sympathetic for the welfare of others. Events such as fireworks, scary stories or movies,

Halloween, and disturbing news can stir great fear in children, causing disturbed sleep.

GRIEF AND DEPRESSION

AURUM METALLICUM

Aurum is a remedy for severe depression, grief, sadness, and despair.
Aurum is highly indicated when suicidal thoughts and impulses are
present, especially after great loss of love, money, possessions, status,
or from wounded honor. The person feels worthless, that there is
nothing to live for. Thinking of suicide may make the person feel better, as well as listening to music. Often a strong religious feeling is
present, with a desire for prayer, meditation, or chanting. Silent grief
is common and may be punctuated by outbursts of anger.

IGNATIA AMARA

Ignatia is an excellent remedy for someone who experiences sudden
grief: from the death of a loved one or beloved pet, the ending of a re-
lationship, or any sudden, overwhelming feeling of emotional loss or
shock. *Ignatia* is more commonly given to women, although many
men have benefited from it as well. Quite often the person feels a
lump in the throat and is given to frequent sighing. The grief may be
silent and restrained but finally releases in a flood of tears and sobbing
that can become hysterical, sometimes a mixture of crying and laugh-
ter. Twitching of the face or around the mouth is often noted. *Ignatia*
is suited to romantic idealists who are sensitive and easily disappointed.

NATRUM MURIATICUM

Natrum is helpful in cases of grief and depression in which the person
prefers to be alone when feeling sad. He or she may be irritated by
consolation and will seldom cry unless completely alone. Usually
from loss of love or disappointment or humiliation, the sadness

is often quite profound; however, the person remains emotionally closed to others to prevent further hurt or rejection. Talking about the feelings is quite difficult. People who need *Natrum* tend to be serious and responsible, often working in helping professions (teacher, counselor, nurse) where they are good listeners but do not risk becoming emotionally vulnerable. They have difficulty letting go of grief and enjoy listening to sad music, while mournful thoughts replay themselves over and over. Bursting headaches and sleeplessness are common among those needing this remedy.

FEVER

Fever represents the body's healthy efforts to fight off disease by creating an internal fire to cleanse the system. Childhood is typically the age of fevers, but adults do get them as well. No matter what the age, unless the fever is extremely high, it should not by itself be cause for great worry, but note that professional advice should be sought for children under six months of age. Often a fever accompanies many types of illnesses, such as earaches, coughs, colds, flu, or childhood illnesses. The aim in treatment is not just removing the fever but bringing the person's overall health back into balance. Therefore, once a remedy is given assessment of the person's progress should be based not on temperature alone but on the general state of health.

After a remedy is given other symptoms may improve before the fever itself drops. In contagious childhood illnesses, a remedy given at the onset will not necessarily prevent the illness from developing but will help minimize discomfort and possibly shorten its course. Whenever a fever is accompanied by other symptoms, consult the appropriate sections of this book for additional remedy choices. (See "Colds, Coughs, and Bronchitis," "Digestive Problems," "Earache," "Influenza," or Part 5.)

The following remedies are indicated during the initial stages of fever.

ACONITE

- Sudden and forceful onset of symptoms after exposure to dry, cold, or windy weather, or after a fright

- During the first twenty-four hours; high fever

- Marked restlessness, anxiety, and fear

- Great thirst

- Face may be red, or alternate between redness and pallor

BELLADONNA

- During the first twenty-four hours

- Sudden and forceful onset of high fever; often worse around 3:00 P.M.

- Face is hot, red, and dry; hot head with cold hands and feet

- Eyes may be red or glazed, with dilated pupils; sensitivity to light

- Tendency to irritability; delirium or hallucinations during sleep

- Little or no thirst

FERRUM PHOSPHORICUM

- Early stages; first twenty-four to forty-eight hours

- No strongly distinguishing symptoms

- Onset is not sudden or intense as with *Aconite* or *Belladonna*

- Fever and flushed cheeks

- Hoarseness or dry cough may be present

The following remedies are indicated in fevers that either develop more gradually or occur further on into an illness.

ARSENICUM ALBUM

- Chilliness, anxiety, and restlessness

- Fever and other symptoms may be worse between midnight and 3:00 A.M.

- Thirst for frequent small sips of water

- Better from warmth and warm drinks

BRYONIA ALBA

- Gradual onset of symptoms, in either warm, humid weather or dry, cold weather

- In influenza with marked body aches

- Worse from all movement; must lie still

- Dryness of all mucous membranes

- Great thirst for cold drinks

- Irritable and grumpy; wants to be left alone

EUPATORIUM PERFOLIATUM

- Flu symptoms with deep, severe aching in bones

- Back feels broken

- Similar to *Bryonia*, except much restlessness; must move to relieve pain

- Very thirsty; desire for iced drinks and ice cream

GELSEMIUM

- Gradual onset of symptoms, especially in warm, humid weather

- Feels dull, drowsy, lethargic; limbs feel heavy

- Heavy, droopy eyelids; face often dusky red; heaviness of tongue

- Flu symptoms with body aches; chills that run up and down back

- Little or no thirst

- Desire to lie still and be left alone

NUX VOMICA

- Fever after overeating, use of alcohol or drugs, or sleep loss

- Headache and digestive symptoms

- Great chilliness from slightest motion or uncovering

- Irritability and oversensitivity to all stimuli

PULSATILLA

- Weepy, mild, and affectionate; craves company and sympathy

- Chilly; worse in a warm room and craves open air

- No thirst

- Changeable symptoms

RHUS TOXICODENDRON

- Fever after exposure to cold, damp weather

- Great restlessness, with body aches and stiffness

- Easily becomes chilled from uncovering

- Flushes of heat alternating rapidly with chill

SULPHUR

- Fever with reddened skin and heat in head and face, similar to *Belladonna*

- Frequent violent flushes of heat, worse at night in bed

- Offensive perspiration, often smelling sour or like sulphur

- When other remedies have not helped

COMMONSENSE MEASURES

- Adequate rest is essential. Limit activity. Quiet bed rest is advised.

- Keeping the head cool and the body warm will help reestablish the right balance of heat in the body. Apply cool washcloths to the forehead and provide adequate fresh air. Keep the rest of the body warmly dressed and/or covered. Avoid cold drinks, because cooling the stomach can direct more heat toward the head.

- Avoid dehydration by giving plenty of room temperature or warm drinks. Hot lemon juice and water is a beneficial drink, especially when the fever is accompanied by any mucus congestion or constipation. Maple syrup may be added for taste and for energy while little or no food is being taken.

- Keep the diet light. Provide small and simple meals. Broth and lightly cooked vegetables are recommended. Partial fasting may also be beneficial.

- To help bring down a very high fever, squeeze the juice of one lemon into a small bowl of tepid water. Immerse a washcloth in it, and sponge the legs and arms in a downward motion. Wipe the face as well. Sponging can be done with plain water if need be.

- Unless complications or clear risks are present, it is far better not to suppress a fever with aspirin or acetaminophen (Tylenol). It's worth noting that aspirin has been associated with Reye's syndrome, and that acetaminophen is known to have risks when taken in excessive doses. When absolutely necessary, acetaminophen is preferred. Fortunately, the majority of uncomplicated fevers in children and adults can be resolved without having to resort to this suppressive measure. The greatest health benefit is derived from allowing nature's healing fire to cleanse the person of illness. The aim is to support the body in reestablishing balance while minimizing the intensity and duration of suffering. Homeopathy can very effectively accomplish this.

- Many parents worry about febrile seizures, but they are not common; though they are frightening when they do occur, complications from them are extremely rare. Fevers are important and necessary events in a child's overall development and immunity, and can be managed safely and effectively with natural home care in most cases. Many parents who have allowed a child's fever to resolve by natural means report that afterward their youngster has gained renewed vigor or crossed a threshold in growth or vitality. Overcoming a fever through one's own healing forces can be strengthening for people of all ages.

SEEK PROFESSIONAL HELP
- If a child's fever rises above 104 degrees

- If a child is under six months of age, seek professional advice in all but the slightest of fevers.

- If there is no response to home treatment within twenty-four hours

- If the fever is associated with a serious illness

- If the fever is accompanied by any of the following: convulsions or seizures, persistent vomiting, visual disturbance, unusual mental confusion, stiff neck, or difficult breathing

FOOD POISONING

Symptoms of food poisoning often include abdominal cramps, nausea, vomiting, and diarrhea. The following remedies are known to bring relief from symptoms that occur after eating contaminated food. (See also "Digestive Problems.")

ARSENICUM ALBUM

- Primary remedy for food poisoning; especially from bad water, meat, or fish

- Burning and cramping pains in stomach

- Burning, offensive-smelling diarrhea that irritates anus

- Nausea with vomiting that burns throat

- Chilly, weak, anxious, and restless

- Cold food and drink are easily vomited

- Better from warmth applied to abdomen and warm drinks

NUX VOMICA

- Nausea, cramps, and painful vomiting

- Marked irritability with nausea; frequent ineffectual attempts to vomit

- Discomfort temporarily relieved by a bowel movement

HEADACHE

Headaches are a common problem and can have a wide variety of causes. Homeopathy can be highly effective in alleviating headaches, and there are many remedies for the different types of headaches. Most common are tension headaches, followed by migraines and those that occur with influenza or other illnesses. Only the most commonly used remedies are included here. (For headaches resulting from head injury, see "Head Injuries and Whiplash.") For relief of acute headache, select one of the following remedies.

ARSENICUM ALBUM

- Burning headache that feels better from cold applications

- Headache associated with food poisoning

- Anxiety and restlessness

- Worse after midnight and from getting chilled

- Better from lying in a darkened room with head slightly elevated

BELLADONNA

- Primary remedy for intense headache that is throbbing, pulsating, or bursting

- Onset often sudden and forceful

- Pupils may be dilated; eyes bloodshot or glazed

- Flushed face; hot head with cold hands and feet

- Worse from heat, sun, light, noise, motion, being jarred, lying flat, bending forward or stooping, cutting the hair

- Better from lying in a quiet, dark room with head elevated, applying firm pressure, bending head backward, closing eyes

BRYONIA ALBA

- Severe aching pain, worse from the slightest motion, even moving eyes

- Pain often begins over left eye and extends over whole head

- Pain increases gradually; dull, heavy, or stitching pains

- Worse from coughing; when constipated

- Irritability, desire to be left alone

- Headache associated with flu, body aches, fever, nausea, or vomiting

- Better from firm pressure and lying on the painful side

GELSEMIUM

- Gradual onset, begins at nape of neck or back of head and spreads to forehead

- General weakness, trembling, drowsiness, and dullness

- Headache may accompany flu or fever

- Head feels very dull and heavy, can hardly hold it up

- Eyelids feel droopy and heavy, can hardly keep them open

- May come on from warm, humid weather or exposure to sun

- Better after urination; from lying with head propped up

IGNATIA AMARA

- Headache associated with grief, sorrow, or disappointment

- Pain feels like a nail being driven into side of head

- Worse from strong emotions, especially unexpressed anger or sadness

- Worse from smoke or strong odors, light, stooping

- Better from lying on the painful side and from warmth

IPECACUANHA

- Severe nausea and vomiting accompany headache

- Bones of head feel crushed or bruised; shooting pains on top of head

- Cold sweat on forehead

- Headache worse from standing; better in open air

IRIS VERSICOLOR

- Marked nausea and vomiting with headache

- Begins with blurred or dimmed vision, or spots before eyes

- Mainly right-sided headache, or alternate sides; forehead, temple, and top of head

- Worse when resting after mental work, from cold air, coughing

- Better from walking in open air, from gentle continued motion

KALI BICHROMICUM

- Headache from sinus infection with congestion and stringy nasal discharge

- Dimmed vision at onset of headache, sight improves as headache worsens

- Much pain at root of nose, better from applying pressure

- Worse from cold, wet weather and lying on the painful side

LACHESIS

- Left-sided headache, or begins on left and moves to right

- Bursting, throbbing pain; sensation of pressing outward

- Pain mostly in forehead, may extend over left eye and root of nose

- Worse on waking in morning, after sleep, from tight collars, strong emotions, heat, before menstrual period, during menopause

- Better from pressure and cool applications, cool air, during any discharges, including menstrual flow

___

NATRUM MURIATICUM

- A primary headache remedy; bursting, squeezing or hammering pain

- Worse in the morning on waking, or from mid-morning to mid-afternoon

- Headache from grief or unexpressed emotions

- Pain often on the right side, or alternating from one location to another

- Pallor, nausea, and vomiting may accompany headache

- Useful in schoolchildren who are serious and introverted

- Worse from heat and sun, prolonged reading or eyestrain

- Better from closing eyes, lying in a darkened room, pressure, cold applications

___

NUX VOMICA

- Headache from overindulgence in food, alcohol, or drugs; stress or mental strain

- Classic hangover; aching at nape of neck and/or forehead

- Nausea and disgust for food during headache

- Worse in the morning from opening eyes, light, odors, noise, cold

- Marked irritability and oversensitivity to all stimuli

- Better from warmth and warm applications, pressure, quiet rest

PHOSPHORUS

- Headache with hunger, or from eating too much sugar

- Chilly, but cold applications and cold air give relief

- Heavy, burning, or pressing pains; often worse on the left side

- Worse from light, warmth, before a thunderstorm, lying on the left side

- Better after sound sleep, eating, cool air or applications

PULSATILLA

- Headache from eating rich or fatty foods; after getting wet or from grief

- Bursting headache with great sense of fullness

- Worse from heat, sun, warm, closed rooms

- Better from open air, gentle motion, cold applications

- Often helpful during puberty and menstrual problems

- Person is sensitive, impressionable, craves affection, cries easily

SANGUINARIA

- Strongly right-sided headache that is throbbing, bursting, or burning

- Often begins in shoulder or neck and settles over right eye or forehead

- Vomiting with headache; sour stomach and indigestion

- Comes and goes with the sun: begins in morning, worse by noon, and eases off by late afternoon

- Worse from jarring, noise, light, odors

- Better after vomiting, from sleep, firm pressure

SPIGELIA

- Strongly left-sided headache; settling in or above left eye and forehead, may extend to back of head

- Severe stitching or shooting pains that fly from one place to another

- Worse in morning, from slightest motion or jarring, noise, smoke, straining or stooping, cold air

- Better from heat, pressure, closing eyes, and lying with head elevated

COMMONSENSE MEASURES

- Depending on the quality of the headache, either cool or warm applications to the head can be helpful. A hot footbath may also give relief in congestive headaches.

- Many headaches are helped by reducing stress. Ways to relieve stress should be suited to each person's individual need and circumstances. Exercise, relaxation techniques, meditation, and artistic activity are among some of the means to reduce stress. Sometimes changes in diet, orientation to work, relationships, or sleep habits are needed. If headaches are a recurrent problem, ask yourself what lifestyle changes might be helpful. Some headaches are hereditary or related to hormonal cycles. In recurrent headaches constitutional treatment is most beneficial.

SEEK PROFESSIONAL HELP

- If there is any combination of the following: marked weakness, visual disturbance, stiff neck, high fever, vomiting, marked drowsiness or dizziness, speech problems

- If headache persists for more than twenty-four hours

- If headaches are a recurrent problem

HEMORRHOIDS

Hemorrhoids (or piles) are a common affliction, especially in the modern, industrialized West. Long hours of sitting and diets high in refined foods are major contributing factors. Although hemorrhoids are often a constitutional problem, homeopathy offers effective short-term relief for acute flare-ups. An external homeopathic ointment may be applied in addition to taking an internal remedy. For long-term improvement a change in diet and exercise, as well as constitutional treatment, may be necessary.

AESCULUS
- Associated with constipation or lower back pain

- Sensation of splinters or sticks in rectum

- Dryness and sense of fullness in rectum

- Pain may last for hours after a bowel movement

ALOE
- Hemorrhoids protrude like a bunch of grapes

- Pain, itching, burning, and heat in rectum

- Open and weak feeling in rectum; easy, involuntary stools

- Better from cold applications

COLLINSONIA

- Constipation and sensation of sticks in rectum

- Marked itching and bleeding

- Worse during menstruation and pregnancy

HAMAMELIS

- Hemorrhoids bleed easily during bowel movements

- Sore, bruised feeling in rectum

IGNATIA AMARA

- Sharp spasms and cutting pains in rectum

- Worse from strong emotion: anger, grief, disappointment

- Pain worse at the end of a bowel movement

NUX VOMICA

- Itching with burning or stinging pain; hemorrhoids with constipation

- For people who are sedentary and/or irritable

- From overuse of laxatives, alcohol, drugs, or coffee

- Better after a bowel movement and from cold bathing

RATANHIA

- Severe pain after a bowel movement, may last for hours

- Pain described as burning, cutting, or like broken glass in rectum

- Hemorrhoids protrude with stool; tendency for cracks in rectum

SULPHUR
- Large, full hemorrhoids that itch terribly

- Irritating moisture in and around rectum; anus may be red and sore

- Worse from standing, drinking beer, warmth; at night

- Better from cold applications

COMMONSENSE MEASURES
- By increasing water intake and fiber in the diet bowel function can be improved, making hemorrhoids less painful. Reducing the intake of refined flour products, and eating more fruits, vegetables, and whole grains will soften stools and relieve pressure on the rectal veins.

- Exercise. Adding more movement to your day can be a big help. If you sit for long periods, get up at frequent intervals and stretch or take a quick, brisk walk when possible.

- *Aesculus* ointment may be applied. Used alone or along with an internal remedy, it often gives substantial relief. *Aesculus* ointment is sometimes sold as a preparation combined with *Hamamelis* and/or *Collinsonia*. Any of these will likely be helpful. For the best effect, apply after a warm sitz bath and before and after each bowel movement. *Calendula* ointment may also be soothing, as well as pads soaked in witch hazel (*Hamamelis*).

SEEK PROFESSIONAL HELP
- If hemorrhoids are severe, persistent, or recurrent

- If rectal bleeding is substantial

INFLUENZA

Typical early symptoms of flu are fever, chills, body aches, and exhaustion. Often sore throat, cold or cough symptoms, or stomach upset may develop. Influenza will usually resolve within one week, though in some cases weakness may linger from several days to several weeks.

The following remedies also appear in other sections of the book pertaining to related symptoms. Please refer to those sections as well to confirm your choice of remedy. (See "Colds, Coughs, and Bronchitis," "Digestive Problems," "Fever," "Headache.")

ACONITE

- Useful during the first twenty-four hours of illness

- (See "Fever")

ARSENICUM ALBUM

- Chilliness, weakness, and exhaustion

- Fever with much restlessness and anxiety

- Burning pains in stomach or throat, nasal discharge, diarrhea

- Thirst for frequent small sips of water

BELLADONNA

- During the first twenty-four hours of illness

- (See "Fever")

BRYONIA ALBA

- Gradual onset of symptoms

- Marked body aches, feels beaten

- Worse from all movement; must lie still

- Often with gastric upset, severe headache, or hard cough

- Dryness of all mucous membranes; much thirst for cold drinks

- Irritable and grumpy; does not want to be disturbed

EUPATORIUM PERFOLIATUM
- Deep, severe aching in bones

- Back feels broken

- Similar to *Bryonia,* except there is much restlessness; must move to relieve pains

- Very thirsty; desire for iced drinks and ice cream

FERRUM PHOSPHORICUM
- During the first twenty-four to forty-eight hours of illness

- (See "Fever")

GELSEMIUM
- Gradual onset of symptoms, especially in warm, humid weather

- Feels dull, drowsy, lethargic; limbs feel heavy and may tremble

- Heavy, droopy eyelids; face often dusky red

- Marked body aches with chills that run up and down back

- Little or no thirst; tongue feels thick and heavy

- Desire to lie still and be left alone

NUX VOMICA
- Great chilliness, worse from slightest motion or uncovering

- Marked headache and digestive symptoms

- Irritability and oversensitivity to all stimuli

OSCILLOCOCCINUM

- During the early stages (first forty-eight hours), when there are few distinguishing symptoms

- May have bursting headache or cough

RHUS TOXICODENDRON

- After exposure to cold, damp weather

- Great restlessness with body aches and stiffness

- During fever easily becomes chilled from uncovering

- Flushes of heat alternating rapidly with chill

COMMONSENSE MEASURES

- See "Fever"

SEEK PROFESSIONAL HELP

- If a serious respiratory condition is present

- If symptoms do not improve

- If diarrhea or great weakness is persistent or severe

INSOMNIA

Everyone experiences insomnia once in a while. For relief of occasional sleeplessness, one of the following remedies can help. Insomnia may be related to another condition or illness, or it can be caused by medications. When insomnia is an ongoing problem, constitutional treatment may be necessary.

ACONITE
- Sleeplessness after a fright or shock, or during onset of fever
- Anxiety; restless sleep with anxious or fearful dreams
- Much tossing and turning

ARNICA MONTANA
- From physical or mental overexertion; too tired to sleep
- Bed feels too hard

ARSENICUM ALBUM
- Indicated when symptoms of illness cause sleeplessness between 12:00 and 2:00 A.M.
- Much restlessness and anxiety, driving the person out of bed
- May have dreams of danger

CHAMOMILLA
- Sleeplessness caused by or resulting in extreme irritability
- Insomnia from physical pains such as toothache or earache
- Helpful during withdrawal from sleeping pills
- Excellent for children's nighttime problems (See "Colic," "Earache," "Teething" in Part 5.)

COFFEA CRUDA
- Sleeplessness from mental excitement; from good news or surprise
- Constant flow of thoughts; racing, uncontrollable thoughts
- Oversensitivity to noise, waking from slightest sound
- Worse from any stimulation to nervous system, from coffee

IGNATIA AMARA

- Sleeplessness with frequent yawning or sighing

- Insomnia associated with grief or sorrow; sobbing during sleep

- Dreams of water or waves; nightmares

KALI PHOSPHORICUM

- Night terrors in children, difficulty falling back to sleep

- Sleeplessness from worry and business troubles; yawning

- Anxious thoughts and sense of dread; restlessness, especially in feet

NUX VOMICA

- Overwork or mental strain; or after overindulgence in food, alcohol, or drugs of any kind

- Worry and marked irritability; waking at 3:00 or 4:00 A.M. and cannot fall back asleep

- Helpful during withdrawal from alcohol, drugs, or sleeping pills

PULSATILLA

- Insomnia after eating rich or fatty foods

- Mild-tempered children who have difficulty sleeping apart from parents

- Fear of being alone, of the dark; clingy and weepy; needs reassurance and sympathy

- Worse in a warm, stuffy room

- Better with window open, from gentle rocking

RHUS TOXICODENDRON
- Great restlessness, much tossing and turning or pacing about
- Difficulty finding a comfortable position
- Pain or stiffness in limbs unless moving them

STRAMONIUM
- Night terrors in children; after a fright
- Wakes in fear with screaming; may recognize no one and remember nothing in the morning
- Fear of being alone in the dark, of animals, death
- Starting or twitching during sleep

STAPHYSAGRIA
- Insomnia from grief, humiliation, or suppressed anger
- Sexual thoughts prevent sleep, may need to masturbate to fall asleep

COMMONSENSE MEASURES
- Establish regular sleeping hours so your body can reliably sense the times for sleeping and waking.
- Avoid eating too close to bedtime, especially rich or cold foods. Allow two hours to digest before retiring.
- Use discretion with alcohol, coffee, chocolate, and many types of drugs (prescription or recreational), especially when used close to bedtime. These substances can prevent sound sleep.
- Avoid watching television too close to bedtime. After viewing give your mind some time to settle back into its natural rhythms. Gentle stretching and deep breathing can be very helpful.

- A hot bath or shower before bed can wash away the tensions of the day and prepare you for sleep.

- A cup of warm milk with honey can be a wonderful natural relaxant before sleep. A one-minute brew of chamomile tea is soothing to the nerves and promotes sleep.

SEEK PROFESSIONAL HELP

- If insomnia is persistent or severe

- If none of the preceding measures helps

JET LAG

For the relief of symptoms of jet lag, select one of the following remedies. If you find one that works well for you, take it as a preventive: Two or three doses within twelve hours of departure. Repeat only as needed thereafter, up to three times daily for no more than three days. (For other problems associated with air travel, see "Motion Sickness.")

ARNICA MONTANA

- Primary remedy for jet lag

- Person feels "beat up," achy, worn out by travel

COCCULUS

- Confusion, spaciness, or dizziness predominate

GELSEMIUM

- Nervousness, trembling, weakness, exhaustion

COMMONSENSE MEASURES

- Avoid alcohol until you feel adjusted to your new location.

- Drink plenty of water before, during, and after the flight.

- Once at your new location, expose yourself to as much daylight as possible each day.

LARYNGITIS

Acute laryngitis is caused by inflammation or overuse of the voice box. The result is hoarseness or loss of the voice. Often laryngitis accompanies other illnesses, such as coughs, colds, or sore throats, or it may be related to allergies. Refer to other relevant sections of this book to confirm your choice of remedy.

ACONITE
- Develops rapidly after exposure to cold weather

- Dry, croupy cough or fever may be present

- Restlessness, anxiety, and fear

ALLIUM CEPA
- Associated with colds that move to larynx and chest

- Colds with profuse, watery nasal discharge

ARNICA MONTANA
- Sudden loss of voice from overuse

CAUSTICUM
- From exposure to dry, cold wind or weather

- Hoarseness or loss of voice from overuse

- Hoarseness worse in the morning

- From anxiety before public speaking or performing

HEPAR SULPHURIS

- Hoarseness with a barking cough, worse in the morning; yellow mucus

- Sore throat with sharp pains when swallowing

- Very chilly and sensitive to drafts and cold

KALI BICHROMICUM

- Colds and coughs with much stringy or ropy yellow mucus

- Worse from cold weather and after eating and drinking

- Better from warmth

PHOSPHORUS

- Hard, dry cough may be present

- Burning pain in throat

- Worse in the evening

- Thirst for cold drinks

RHUS TOXICODENDRON

- From overuse speaking or singing

- Worse when beginning to speak, improves with continued use

COMMONSENSE MEASURES

- Rest the voice as much as possible.

- Warm drinks such as herbal teas with honey and lemon are soothing.

- Gargling with sage tea often helps.

- Chamomile steam inhalation (see page 115), a warm compress on neck and throat, and use of a humidifier are other helpful measures.

SEEK PROFESSIONAL HELP

- If laryngitis is persistent, severe, or painful

- If the preceding measures do not help

MOTION SICKNESS

Travel can be very unpleasant for those afflicted with motion sickness. A well-selected homeopathic remedy not only will greatly alleviate symptoms once they occur but also may be taken as a preventive before traveling. Select one remedy that best suits the overall condition. As a preventive (if you anticipate motion sickness), give two or three doses of the remedy on the day before travel and once again an hour before the journey begins. Repeat every two to three hours only as needed (if symptoms are present).

BORAX

- Nausea and vomiting

- Especially worse from downward motion

COCCULUS

- Severe nausea, vomiting; with dizziness (vertigo)

- Increased salivation

- Vertigo, especially from watching moving objects

- Sight or smell of food greatly aggravates nausea

- Desire to lie down

- Worse from becoming cold and from noise

NUX VOMICA
- Nausea with terrible headache; faintness

- Painful gagging and retching

- Chilly and constipated

- Aggravated by coffee, tobacco, and food

PETROLEUM
- Nausea and dizziness

- Faintness and pallor

- Empty, hungry feeling relieved by eating small amounts

- Cold perspiration

- Pain in back of head or neck

- Increased salivation

TABACUM
- Severe nausea with vomiting

- Pallor and coldness, with cold perspiration

- Need for cool, fresh air

- Faintness or giddiness

- Tight sensation around head, like a band

- Especially aggravated by cigarette smoke

- Closing eyes relieves symptoms a bit

COMMONSENSE MEASURES
- Whether traveling by car, airplane, or boat, you can help minimize the severity of discomfort by ensuring adequate fresh air,
avoiding smoke or food odors, and keeping eyes focused on dis-
tant, nonmoving objects. If traveling by car, frequent stops can
be helpful. Sipping ginger tea or sucking a piece of candied ginger may also help to reduce nausea.

SINUS INFECTION

Homeopathic medicines can be very effective in treating symptoms of
acute sinus infection, or sinusitis. Usually a sinus infection begins
with a simple cold or allergy that produces sinus congestion. When
bacteria spreads in the sinuses, inflammation increases and infection
develops. Common symptoms include yellow-green discharge, facial
pain and pressure, headache, fever, and fatigue. Refer also to other
relevant sections of the book, such as "Colds, Coughs, and Bronchitis," "Fever," or "Headache," to make the best remedy selection.

BELLADONNA
- Much throbbing pain, frontal headache; often worse on the
right side

- Fever may be present (see "Fever" for more indications)

- Pain severe when stooping or bending and from jarring

HEPAR SULPHURIS
- Advanced, painful sinusitis with blockage and much thick yellow mucus

- Discharge worse from exposure to cold air; foul or cheesy odor of discharge

- Great sensitivity to pain; bursting headache, scalp painful to touch

KALI BICHROMICUM

- A primary remedy for sinus infection

- Thick, stringy, ropy, or gluey nasal discharge; postnasal drip

- Discharge yellow or yellow-green and difficult to expel; complete obstruction of sinuses

- Marked pain and fullness at root of nose, better from pressing there

LYCOPODIUM

- Right-sided sinusitis with nasal discharge

- Nostrils may become crusted and irritated

- Marked obstruction, worse at night while sleeping

MERCURIUS VIVUS

- A primary remedy for advanced sinus infection; greenish discharge

- Discharge may be acrid and offensive smelling; offensive breath

- Tongue often coated grayish; marked increased salivation

- Pain in facial bones and in roots of teeth, worse at night

PULSATILLA

- Bland yellowish or greenish nasal discharge with frontal headache

- Worse in a warm room, from stooping, rising after rest, lying with head low

- Better from cool or open air, gentle continued motion, lying with head propped up, or binding head

- Thirstlessness, even with a dry mouth

SILICA

- Chronically obstructed nose after a cold; postnasal drip

- Bursting headache, often settles over or in one eye; dizziness

- Pain worse from cold weather, light, noise, and moving head

- Very chilly; cold perspiration of feet

SPIGELIA

- Left-sided sinusitis with sharp, stabbing pains in forehead or behind left eye

- Worse from exposure to cold, damp weather

COMMONSENSE MEASURES

- Steam inhalation from a hot shower or a chamomile steam inhalation (see page 115) can be very soothing, even when the nose is completely obstructed.

- Drink plenty of hot lemon water (one lemon squeezed into a tall glass of hot water) with a pinch of cayenne pepper added.

- Nasal douching with salt water often helps open sinuses. A neti pot, used in Ayurvedic medicine from India, is a convenient device for nasal douching.

- Avoid wheat and dairy products, since they tend to exacerbate mucus production.

- See Commonsense Measures under "Colds, Coughs, and Bronchitis."

SEEK PROFESSIONAL HELP
- If symptoms are severe or prolonged

- If the preceding measures do not help

SKIN PROBLEMS

The skin is the largest organ of the human body and is often where an internal imbalance finds its expression. Rashes, boils, pimples, itching, and other skin symptoms should be seen as the body's best attempts to eliminate or clear out such imbalances. The skin is the most peripheral organ of the physical body, and thus the last hurdle to overcome in the process of restoring health. Because of this, *it is especially important that skin symptoms not be suppressed or driven backward, deeper into the body,* by the use of steroids or other treatments that tend to mask symptoms. The ideal is to heal from the inside out while strengthening one's resistance to future illness. Chronic or recurring problems such as acne, eczema, and psoriasis should ultimately be addressed by homeopathic constitutional care or other nonsuppressive natural measures.

BOILS
Boils occur when a person is susceptible to infection. Often painful, boils are inflamed skin eruptions filled with pus. They usually appear on the face, neck, or buttocks and are hot, red, and swollen. Eventually each boil comes to a head, releases pus, and heals quickly; sometimes boils do not open, and the fluid is absorbed into the body as the boil heals. Homeopathy can assist the healing process. Select from among the following remedies.

ARSENICUM ALBUM

- Boils characterized by burning pain that feels better from warm applications

- Other general characteristics of *Arsenicum* (see Part 6)

BELLADONNA

- Early stage of boils, most effective before much pus has formed

- Hot, red, angry-looking boils; pulsating or throbbing pain

HEPAR SULPHURIS

- Boils extremely painful from slightest touch

- Often slow in coming to a head

- Boils that develop from a small cut or scrape

- Person is chilly and much bothered by cold air

HYPERICUM

- Very painful boils with sharp, shooting pains

- In boils where there is no discharge of pus

SILICA

- Boils slow to heal, even after pus has drained

- Boils that develop from a small cut or scrape (*Hepar sulphuris*)

- Similar to *Hepar sulphuris*, but pain and sensitivity to touch are not as severe

- Boils leave cystic lumps when mostly healed

SULPHUR

- Soon after crops of boils heal, new ones appear; recurrent boils

- Generally skin is rough or unhealthy and boils tend to heal slowly

- Markedly red, hot boils; often on buttocks

TARENTULA CUBENSIS

- Boils very large and purple or bluish purple

- Intense burning and stinging pain, worse at night

COMMONSENSE MEASURES

- Soak or apply a hot compress to encourage the boils to come to a head and drain. Very painful boils may be soaked in hot water to which *Hypericum* mother tincture has been added.

- Apply *Calendula* or Hypercal ointment to help heal the skin once boils have opened and drained.

SEEK PROFESSIONAL HELP

- If boils are a recurrent problem

- If fever or glandular swelling is present

- If no improvement is seen within two days

HIVES

Hives (nettle rash or urticaria) are an allergic reaction characterized by flat or raised red blotches on the skin. They usually feel itchy and hot; in some cases swelling may be pronounced. Hives are caused by a variety of influences: foods such as shellfish or strawberries, allopathic medications, insect bites, overheating, or exposure to sun. Many food additives can cause hives as well. A homeopathic remedy can work quickly to stabilize the allergic reaction and reduce discomfort.

APIS MELLIFICA

- Raised red blotches that feel markedly worse from warmth of any kind

- Skin feels swollen and tense, as if it would burst; marked itching and stinging

- Insect bites and stings; reactions to eating shellfish or strawberries

- Allergic swelling of lips, face, or around eyes

- Worse when overheated: after exertion, exposure to sun, at night in bed, from fever

NUX VOMICA

- Hives with digestive complaints; food or drug allergies

- Itching with burning; chill from uncovering

- Irritability and impatience may be present

PULSATILLA

- After eating rich or fatty foods, often accompanied by diarrhea

- In some cases where menstruation is delayed

- Worse from warmth and being in a closed room; better in open air

RHUS TOXICODENDRON

- From cold air, getting wet, or during fever

- Restlessness

- Itching relieved by applying very hot water

SULPHUR

- From food or drug allergies; during fever

- Great heat and itchiness, worse from warmth, exercise, and at night

- Better in cool air

URTICA URENS

- True nettle rash; red and raised hives; itching and burning

- Prickling, sunburned, or scalded sensation

- Violent itching with desire to rub

- From eating shellfish or strawberries

- Worse from warmth, exertion, any heat

COMMONSENSE MEASURES

- Cool applications usually afford some relief.

SEEK PROFESSIONAL HELP

- If there is swelling in the mouth or throat

- If breathing is impeded or difficult

- If there is a history of severe reactions

POISON OAK OR IVY

Indigenous to the American continent, poison oak and poison ivy are well known for the rash that contact with the plants produces. Each plant causes virtually identical reactions on the skin. The oils from *Rhus toxicodendron* typically cause intense itching and some degree of blistering and can easily be spread to other parts of the body. Unfortunately, people who get the rash repeatedly often find that it worsens with each occurrence. Conventional treatment consists of topical or systemic steroids, which are suppressive and should be avoided. Their continued or repeated use can lead to more severe reactions in future contacts with the plant. Most cases will resolve on their own within about ten days; however, when symptoms cause considerable suffering and distress, homeopathic treatment will often give welcome relief.

Give a 12C or 30C potency three to five times per day depending on the severity of symptoms for two or three days, less often as symptoms improve. If after five doses there is no change, discontinue and try another remedy.

ANACARDIUM

- Intense itching that becomes worse from scratching, with burning and stinging

- Worse from warmth, but relieved by scalding hot water

- Blisters and pustules that are yellow with red around the edges

- Often the left side of the body is more strongly affected

APIS MELLIFICA

- Great swelling and heat in affected areas

- Itching, burning, and stinging, worse from heat of any kind

- Minimal blistering, but marked redness and swelling

- Often occurs on face or around eyes

- Better from applying cold water or ice

CROTON TIGLIUM

- Severe itching, skin becomes thickened

- Clusters of blisters that become larger and exude yellow fluid

- Face and genital region often affected

GRAPHITES

- Advanced rash with thick yellow discharge like honey; many thick crusts

- Irresistible itching; must scratch until it's raw, which gives relief

- Itching and burning worse from heat of bed

- Often affects bends of elbows and knees, any folds in skin

RHUS TOXICODENDRON (THE POISON IVY PLANT ITSELF)

- Intense itching, burning, tingling, or prickling sensations

- Rash causes great restlessness

- Itching much worse from scratching; worse from getting wet and cold air

- Scalding hot water gives relief

- Small or large blisters surrounded by very red skin

- Eruptions may spread in a linear fashion

SEPIA

- Blisters produce an irritating discharge that burns skin

- Skin often yellowish, with eruptions in folds

- Worse in the evening; from cold air

- Better from scratching, warmth

SULPHUR

- Intense, irresistible itching with much burning; better from cold applications

- Must scratch until skin is raw and bloody, which gives relief

- Tendency to a moist rash that is easily infected

- Blisters and pustules surrounded by deep red skin

- Much worse at night, from heat of bed, sweating, any heat

- Often affects the left side; at bends or folds of skin

COMMONSENSE MEASURES

- Cleaning the plant's oils from the skin is essential to prevent further spreading. Tecnu and Fels Naptha are both excellent cleansers especially for this purpose. Wash gently two or three times per day using tepid water.

- An oatmeal bath such as Aveeno can give much relief of itching and may be taken several times per day if needed. Take care that the plant's oils have been well removed before immersion in the bath.

- In relatively dry forms of the rash (those that are not excessively weepy), green clay may be applied to affected areas. (Green-clay powder is available at most health food stores.) Make a medium-thin paste by adding a little water and a few drops of *Calendula* tincture to 1 tablespoon of the powder and apply a thin layer over the area. This helps prevent spreading of the rash and isolates the itch. Leave it on most of the day and reapply after each cleaning if you wish.

- *Aloe vera* gel gives cooling relief of burning pain and can assist the healing of the skin after blisters have broken. *Calendula* spray or ointment may also be used.

SEEK PROFESSIONAL HELP

- If marked pus, swelling, fever, severe redness, or red streaks appear

WARTS

Warts are caused by a viral infection that results in overgrowth of skin cells. Some people are extremely susceptible to the viruses that cause warts, while others are not at all. This underlying predisposition is a factor often best addressed through constitutional homeopathic treatment. However, the following remedies are known to be successful and may be tried over a limited time as shorter-term treatments. If recurrence is a problem and if warts are troublesome, seek professional care. Give a 6C potency twice per day for two to four weeks. Discontinue as soon as there is improvement. If there is no change after two weeks, try another remedy.

ANTIMONIUM CRUDUM

- Plantar warts on soles of feet

- Warts are hardened, callused or horny, and have a smooth surface

CAUSTICUM

- Warts appear primarily on face, eyelids, and fingers near the nails

- Soft, fleshy warts

DULCAMARA

- Warts on backs of hands

- Hard, smooth, or fleshy warts

NITRIC ACID

- Warts on upper lip, genitals, and anus

- Cauliflower-like warts that itch, sting, or have sticking pains

- Warts often of irregular shape, soft and tend to bleed

SEPIA

- Large brown or black warts with hairs growing out of them

- More often occurring in women

THUJA

- May appear anywhere on the body

- Common sites: back of head, chin, genitals, and anus

- Warts are soft and cauliflower-like, and tend to ooze and bleed

COMMONSENSE MEASURES

- Apply *Thuja* mother tincture or ointment on rising in the morning and again before going to sleep.

SURGERY

Whether in the case of a minor operation or in major surgery, homeopathic remedies can help minimize the physical and emotional shock from such procedures and can significantly speed healing.

Arnica is highly recommended as the remedy of first choice for a wide range of surgery situations. In many cases where *Arnica* has been given, doctors are amazed at how quickly their patients recover and how little pain medication is needed. As a general guideline, give a 30C potency three times during the twenty-four hours before surgery. Repeat in the same manner postoperatively for up to three days. As a rule, the deeper or more invasive the surgery, the higher the potency needed. For a major operation, such as hip replacement, give *Arnica* 200C three times within twenty-four hours before surgery and afterward three times daily for up to three days. Give other remedies before surgery in the same manner where indicated, and otherwise afterward as needed according to the first aid dosage guidelines in Part 3.

ACONITE

- Marked anxiety, fear, and restlessness before or after surgery

- Great fear of death

ARNICA MONTANA

- Primary remedy for the physical trauma of surgery

- Much soreness, aching, and bruised feeling

BELLIS PERENNIS

- Useful especially before or after deep abdominal or pelvic surgery

- Trauma to soft organs of abdomen; may be marked swelling

HYPERICUM

- Give before and after surgery in areas rich in nerves: spine, head, hands, or feet

- Pains are sharp or shooting

- Dental or oral surgery with sharp or shooting pains

PHOSPHORUS

- Helpful for symptoms that may follow general anesthesia: confusion, fearfulness, nausea, and vomiting

STAPHYSAGRIA

- Pain in incision; poorly healing incision

- Pain remains after surgery to genitals

THROAT COMPLAINTS

Sore throats and infections are common problems for people of all ages. When resistance is low, a bacterial or viral infection can result. A simple sore throat may remain just that or can accompany related symptoms such as fever, malaise, swollen glands, or tonsillitis. Whether a throat inflammation is caused by a virus or bacteria, homeopathy can be highly effective because it aims to raise overall resistance by treating the person, not the disease (or virus or bacteria). There are some instances where the use of antibiotics may be warranted to offset risk factors in streptococcal infections (strep throat). See the end of this section for further comments about strep.

Because other ailments such as fever, cold, and flu can accompany sore throat, you may wish to refer to these or other sections of the book when appropriate to help confirm your remedy choice.

The following three remedies are often indicated during the initial stages of throat inflammations.

ACONITE

- Sudden and forceful onset after exposure to cold or to dry, cold wind; or after a fright

- During the first twenty-four hours; high fever

- Marked restlessness, anxiety, and fear

- Great thirst with fever

- Face may be red, or may alternate between redness and pallor

BELLADONNA

- Primary remedy during the initial stage of sore throat or tonsillitis, especially in children; symptoms often right-sided

- Sudden and forceful onset of symptoms, with high fever

- Throat and tonsils are bright red, with swelling and/or white patches

- Burning pain, strong desire to swallow, though causes much pain

- Face is hot, red, and dry; hot head with cold hands and feet

- Worse from slightest touch of throat, swallowing liquids

- Little or no thirst; may desire lemonade

FERRUM PHOSPHORICUM

- Early stages; first twenty-four to forty-eight hours

- Inflamed tonsils or sore throat; hot, red, and swollen

- Fever and slightly flushed cheeks

- No other strongly distinguishing symptoms

- Onset not sudden or intense as with *Aconite* or *Belladonna*

- Hoarseness or dry cough may be present

The following remedies are indicated for a range of throat inflammations that either develop more gradually or are indicated further into the illness.

APIS MELLIFICA

- Very swollen tonsils or swollen sensation in sore throat, with stinging pains

- Constrictive sensation, with burning and stinging; uvula may be swollen

- Throat pain even when *not* swallowing; sensation of a fish bone

- Much worse from heat of any kind, better from cold drinks and ice

ARSENICUM ALBUM

- Burning throat pain, better from warm food and drinks; worse from cold

- Milky white coating of tongue

- Small ulcers or sores in throat

- Symptoms often right-sided

GELSEMIUM

- Symptoms appear slowly, worsening over days

- Marked throat pain, extending into ear on swallowing

- Great weakness, heaviness, and dull feeling

- Fever, chill, and flulike symptoms; a remedy for mononucleosis

HEPAR SULPHURIS

- A primary remedy for more advanced inflammations with pus; ulcers or abscesses

- Very sharp, splinterlike pains, often extending to ear on swallowing

- Very chilly and oversensitive to pain; worse from anything cold; better from warm drinks

- Extremely irritable

IGNATIA AMARA

- Better while swallowing foods; worse from empty swallowing

- Sensation of a lump in throat; constant urge to swallow

- May be associated with unexpressed strong emotions or grief

LACHESIS

- Left-sided throat inflammations and tonsillitis, may spread from left to right

- Tonsils, throat, and/or uvula may be swollen and dark red or purple

- Worse from warm drinks, during sleep, on waking in morning

- Neck very sensitive to touch; constricting sensation; difficulty swallowing liquids

LYCOPODIUM

- Right-sided throat inflammations, may spread from right to left

- Worse from cold drinks; better from warm drinks

- Symptoms worse between 4:00 and 8:00 P.M.

MERCURIUS VIVUS

- Often more advanced inflammations, frequently with sores and ulcers

- Great sensitivity to both heat and cold; narrow comfort range

- Constant urge to swallow; increased saliva, especially at night, drooling on pillow

- Pus on tonsils, offensive breath, metallic taste in mouth

- All symptoms worse at night; night sweats

MERCURIUS IODATUS RUBER

- Mercurius vivus symptoms that are strongly left-sided

MERCURIUS IODATUS FLAVUS

- Mercurius vivus symptoms that are strongly right-sided

PHYTOLACCA

- Often right-sided pain, with sharp pain into ear on swallowing

- Tonsils swollen, dark, or purplish, with much burning pain; worse from warm drinks

- Painfully swollen glands of neck

- Pain in root of tongue, especially when tongue is protruded

RHUS TOXICODENDRON

- Symptoms after exposure to cold, wet weather or from straining voice

- Tongue often coated white, with tip red, like a triangle

- Pain on first swallowing, better with successive swallows

- Often with cold or flu, or stiffness of muscles and joints

SULPHUR

- A remedy to try after other remedies have not helped

- Marked burning pain relieved by cold drinks

- Swollen tonsils, offensive breath, bright red lips

COMMONSENSE MEASURES

- Dress warmly in cold weather. The throat is often the gateway to other cold-weather illnesses. Layer clothing, and wear a turtleneck or scarf to protect the throat. Keep the head and feet warm and dry. Protecting the throat can prevent colds, flus, and chest conditions.

- At the first signs of illness, drink hot lemon water with a pinch of cayenne pepper: one tall glass at bedtime and once again in the morning on rising. No food should be taken within one hour for best effect. Hot lemon and honey drinks can be very sooth-ing. In general, increase the intake of warm, clear fluids.

- Keep the diet light, warming, and simple.

- Extra vitamin C is helpful, especially at the outset: 500 mg four times per day.

- Drink echinacea tea or tincture added to herbal tea; suck zinc lozenges with slippery elm.

- Use a saltwater gargle: 1 teaspoon of sea salt dissolved in 1 cup of hot water. Add 10 to 20 drops of *Calendula* tincture to the solu-tion and gargle three times per day. In infections that produce yellow mucus or spots on the throat or tonsils, add 10 drops each of *Goldenseal* tincture (*Hydrastis canadensis*) and *Calendula* tinc-ture to the gargle solution.

SEEK PROFESSIONAL HELP

- If pain or swelling is severe or impedes breathing or swallowing

- If marked throat inflammation does not improve in a child within forty-eight hours, or in an adult after four days

- If the person has a history of rheumatic fever

- If there are whitish or yellowish spots or deposits on the tonsils or throat

- In cases of streptococcal throat infection (strep throat), conven-tional medicine in the United States considers the use of anti-biotics necessary because of the risk of developing rheumatic fever or kidney inflammation. Though rare, these complications do pose enough of a risk to be weighed carefully by some indi-viduals when choosing treatment. But not all strep-type infec-tions will rage out of control without antibiotics. Many strep throats go undiagnosed and resolve on their own. In the United Kingdom, throat infections are seldom cultured and are simply called sore throats or tonsillitis; indeed the term *strep throat* does not exist in the popular vocabulary there.

Homeopathic remedies can be highly effective in treating people with strep and other throat infections, and can over time strengthen the natural resistance to infection. A remedy may be given in conjunction with commonsense measures while awaiting the results of a throat culture or along with antibiotics should either become necessary. Discuss the risks with your family doctor. Especially where there is a family history of problems related to strep, prompt medical attention is advised. Constitutional homeopathic treatment is highly recommended if throat infections are a recurrent problem.

TOOTH PAIN

Homeopathic remedies have wide success in the treatment of a variety of dental conditions. In most cases a visit to the dentist is warranted and a remedy can be taken before as well as after dental treatment. For relief of acute tooth pain, select from the following remedies.

ACONITE
- Sudden, intense toothache causing much anxiety, distress, and fear

- After exposure to cold, dry wind

- After fright or shock

ARNICA MONTANA
- Primary remedy for injuries to teeth

- Excellent after dental extractions or other procedures

- May be given before (and after) dental work to prevent pain

- Sore, aching, bruised feeling

BELLADONNA

- Sudden pains in teeth; intense throbbing pain; cavities

- Red and swollen gums

- Pains often right-sided

CHAMOMILLA

- Primary remedy for children's teething pain (see "Teething")

- Severe pains, worse at night in bed, from cold air, drinking coffee

- Pain from a cavity or cracked tooth, often causing great irritability and anger

COFFEA CRUDA

- Restlessness, agitation, and insomnia from toothache

- Severe jerking and tearing pains, better from holding cold water in mouth

HEPAR SULPHURIS

- Cavities, infected gums, and abscesses, causing intense, sharp pains

- Severely sensitive to the slightest touch, to anything cold (air, food, drinks)

- Extremely irritable

HYPERICUM

- Tooth injuries with sharp, shooting pains

- After dental work when sharp, shooting pains are present

- May be given before dental work when such pains are anticipated

MERCURIUS VIVUS

- Cavities and infections with foul breath and increased salivation

- Great and painful sensitivity in teeth to both heat and cold

- Metallic taste in mouth

- Throbbing pains, worse at night; may extend to face or into ear

STAPHYSAGRIA

- Cavities, especially in children; crumbling teeth

- Severe pain from the slightest touch, throbbing or tearing

- Pain worse from cold air, cold drinks

COMMONSENSE MEASURES

- Good oral hygiene is important for prevention of tooth and gum disease.

- Topical application of Ipsab herbal gum treatment is very effective in soothing superficial gum soreness. For abscesses and other deeper problems, a visit to the dentist is warranted.

SEEK PROFESSIONAL HELP

- Visit the dentist in all but the most superficial conditions.

WOMEN'S AILMENTS

Women's ailments encompass a broad range of conditions. An entire volume could be devoted to the subject; indeed quite a few books have been written on this topic alone. This section will discuss ailments that are most common and well suited to acute treatment: bladder infection, premenstrual syndrome (PMS) and menstrual cramps, and vaginitis. These and many other ailments particular to women are cyclical or tend to be recurrent and are thus often best suited to constitutional treatment. It should be stressed that the following recommendations are for self-treatment of occasional ailments and that frequently recurring, severe, or chronic problems require professional care. For a broader range of information on homeopathic women's health care, see "Suggested Readings."

BLADDER INFECTION

A bladder infection, or cystitis, can be very uncomfortable. It is more common in women and girls, because bacteria can more easily enter the bladder due to a shorter urethra. Homeopathic remedies have proven very effective in alleviating the discomfort of bladder infections. If recurrence is a problem, seek constitutional treatment.

Select one of the following remedies and give one dose every one to four hours depending on the severity of symptoms. Repeat the remedy less often as symptoms improve. If symptoms do not improve after three or four doses, try another remedy.

ACONITE
- Symptoms appear suddenly after exposure to cold or fright

- Anxiety and fear with urge to urinate

- Pressure and burning

APIS MELLIFICA

- Marked stinging and burning pain, especially at the beginning of urination

- Similar to *Cantharis*; restless feeling

- Worse from heat and at night; better from cold

CANTHARIS

- Intense burning pain with urination; urine scalds and burns as it passes

- Constant urge to urinate but can pass only a few drops

- Person may shriek with pain while urinating; restlessness and frantic feeling

- Pains throughout bladder, relieved for a short time after urination

- Blood may be passed with urine

NUX VOMICA

- Constant urge to urinate but can pass only a small amount

- Spasms in bladder

- Person may be irritable, agitated, and oversensitive to all stimuli

- Urge to move bowels during urination

- Worse from being chilled, alcohol, coffee

PULSATILLA

- Sudden, intense urges to urinate, must rush to the bathroom

- The more she holds it in, the more painful it is

- Involuntary spurting of urine from coughing, sneezing, or laughing

- Urine may contain mucus or blood

SARSAPARILLA

- Marked burning pain at the end of urination, as the last drops are passed

- Chill during urination

- Symptoms worse from cold, damp weather and before or during menstrual period

STAPHYSAGRIA

- Bladder infection after intercourse; "honeymoon" cystitis

- Burning and frequent urge to urinate, unfinished feeling

COMMONSENSE MEASURES

- Preventive measures include careful hygiene in the bathroom; always wipe from front to back.

- Always promptly heed the urge to urinate.

- When symptoms first appear, drink lots of clear fluids; unsweetened cranberry juice is helpful; eliminate all other fruit juices, sugar, and caffeine from the diet.

- Other helpful measures include drinking herbal teas: dandelion, nettle, sarsaparilla, or uva ursi (bearberry).

SEEK PROFESSIONAL HELP

- If symptoms do not improve within forty-eight hours

- If there is a history of kidney disease

- If urine looks bloody or reddish brown

- If symptoms are severe or accompanied by any of the following: fever, headache, vomiting, pain in the kidney area (in the back above lower ribs), or swelling of the abdomen, face, or ankles

PREMENSTRUAL SYNDROME (PMS) AND MENSTRUAL CRAMPS

Homeopathic remedies can be very effective in relieving the physical discomforts and emotional shifts that many women experience around their menstrual periods. Cramps, bloating, breast swelling and tenderness, fatigue, water retention, and headaches are common complaints. Many women also become more prone to emotional changes, feeling more irritable and short-tempered, weepy, moody, or generally more sensitive and vulnerable. The following homeopathic remedies can help with many of these complaints. One dose may be given every two hours during intense symptoms, or every three to four hours for moderate to mild symptoms. Stop the remedy when there is improvement, and repeat only as needed. If there is no change after three or four doses, try a different remedy. You may wish to refer to other relevant sections of the book, such as "Headache" or "Abdominal Pain," to confirm your choice of remedy.

BELLADONNA

- Intense bearing-down or cramping pains that come and go suddenly

- Headache, usually pulsating or throbbing, with heat and flushed face

- Worse from motion, especially jarring or stepping

- Blood is bright red; may be mixed with dark clots

CALCAREA CARBONICA

- General sense of weakness and fatigue; clumsiness

- Headache, anxiety, and breast swelling and tenderness; nausea

- Chilly; sweaty, often in genital area

- Tendency to heavy bleeding and vaginitis

CIMICIFUGA RACEMOSA

- Cramping, shooting pains that dart from one side of the body to the other

- Menstrual cramps worsen as flow increases

- Overwhelmed feeling; dull, gloomy, or hazy feeling with headache

- Talkative and sometimes hysterical

COLOCYNTHIS

- Intense cramps similar to *Magnesia phosphorica*

- Great restlessness and irritability; impatient and easily angered

- Better from bending double; hard pressure

IGNATIA AMARA

- Menstruation brings on grief and sadness; emotional vulnerability

- Irritability from the slightest contradiction

- Spasmodic pains; hysteria, feeling of lump in throat, sighing

LACHESIS

- Irritable, talkative, sharp-tongued, sarcastic, suspicious, jealous

- Bloating, headache, severe cramping

- All symptoms relieved as soon as or after menstrual flow begins

- Pains worse on left side, worse during sleep or upon waking

MAGNESIA PHOSPHORICA

- Cramps relieved by bending double

- Better from firm pressure, hot applications (hot water bottle), hot drinks

NUX VOMICA

- Cramping pains with frequent urge for a bowel movement; nausea

- Irritable, impatient, competitive, argumentative

PULSATILLA

- Cramps in women who are mild, gentle, and moody; tend to weep easily

- Nausea and bloating often pronounced, water retention worse during warm weather

- Tendency for irregular or changeable menstrual periods

- Generally worse in a warm, closed room; better from open air

SEPIA

- Exhaustion, bloating, cramps, and constipation common

- Moodiness and marked irritability; short-tempered, sad

- Critical; indifference or aversion to family members; desire to be alone

- Vigorous exercise and dancing often alleviate many symptoms

COMMONSENSE MEASURES

- In anticipation of menstrual discomforts, try to reduce the influence of known stressors when possible, and allow time for extra rest if needed. In many traditional cultures it is the custom for women to set aside some of their routine activities during menstruation. Though this idea may seem impractical, it is worth viewing the time of bleeding as also a time of cleansing and renewal, and that it may be helpful to consider modification of activities.

VAGINITIS

Vaginitis, or vaginal infection, is an inflammation of the vagina that creates abnormal discharge and itching or burning pains. The infection can be caused by the presence of a number of bacteria or, most commonly, an overabundance of a normally occurring yeast called *Candida albicans.* In the homeopathic approach to vaginitis, the unique symptoms of the individual woman, rather than particular causative agents, determine the choice of remedy.

BORAX
- Burning vaginal discharge; thick, clear, and gelatinous, like the white of an egg

- Often occurs midway between menstrual periods

CALCAREA CARBONICA
- Milky white or thick yellow discharge, causing intense itching

- Often occurs midway between menstrual periods or shortly before menses

- In women who tend to be chilly, fair-skinned, and overweight

GRAPHITES
- Whitish, thin, watery, acrid discharge; sometimes with backache; much itching

- In women who are overweight; dullness or anxiety in the morning on waking

HYDRASTIS
- Profuse yellow, stringy discharge

KREOSOTE
- Much itching and burning; yellow discharge that smells like rye bread
- Discharge causes much irritation and even swelling in vaginal lips and surrounding tissues
- Severe burning when urine touches irritated parts
- General weakness and irritability

PULSATILLA
- Bland, nonirritating discharge, may be white, yellow, or greenish
- Often needed for vaginitis during pregnancy
- In women who are mild, gentle, and moody; tending to weep easily; often thirstless
- Worse from heat or in closed rooms; better in open air

SEPIA
- Offensive-smelling discharge, milky white or more often yellow
- Dragging or heavy feeling in pelvic area
- Exhaustion, irritability, depression, and constipation common

COMMONSENSE MEASURES
- Careful hygiene makes for good prevention as well as proper care during vaginitis.

- Homeopathic suppositories are also available, and are often helpful, though trying an individualized internal remedy is a preferable first option.

- A homemade garlic suppository is helpful to many women. Peel one clove of garlic, leaving the thin outer membrane intact. Wrap in a small piece of sterile gauze and insert into the vagina. It may be left in for up to twelve hours and works well in conjunction with a homeopathic remedy or alone.

- Douching with yogurt is also helpful to many women. Use an "organic-quality" plain yogurt that is high in lactobacillus cultures.

SEEK PROFESSIONAL HELP

- If fever or severe pelvic pain accompanies vaginitis

- If vaginal infections are severe, persistent, or recurring

PART 5

CHILDHOOD CONDITIONS

A WORD ABOUT VACCINES

Routine childhood vaccination has become increasingly debated over recent years. Clear evidence shows that vaccines have damaged many children's health. Vaccines pose risks ranging from reactions that produce a lowered resistance to common infections, to seizures and serious physical and mental handicaps, to even death, and ought to be investigated by every parent. Yet the majority of children show no apparent health problems after being vaccinated, and they are protected from certain diseases to a measurable degree. Parents seeking a more natural approach to strengthening their children's immunity face a difficult decision.

Today's American children are more likely to receive a greater number of vaccines than their parents did, at more frequent intervals, and starting at an earlier age. In deeply altering the immature and delicate immune systems of babies and children, vaccines are bound to produce some negative consequences in a percentage of the population. For vaccinated children, the increased risk of their developing chronic diseases emerging in adulthood have not been adequately researched. However, some studies have charted a connection between the advent of vaccines and the decline of acute illnesses with a parallel increase in chronic diseases during the twentieth century.

The suppression of childhood illness with conventional interventions gives little opportunity for a child's immune system to overcome illness on its own. Routine vaccination combined with liberal use of antibiotics and fever-reducing drugs such as acetaminophen create a sterile environment where the child's own healing forces cannot grow in step with the other aspects of his development. Acute inflammatory illnesses can actually strengthen the immune system as a child moves through the sequence of developmental milestones. Many common childhood illnesses can be managed effectively with natural means such as those provided in this book, or with the help of a professional homeopath or other natural health care provider.

The education of the immune system can be compared to the process of a child learning to walk. A child may repeatedly stumble and fall, perhaps scraping his knee or getting a few bruises. As he learns the parameters of his environment, about gravity, balance, and which movements work well and not so well, he becomes a better walker. He would not learn to be autonomous if someone were to hold on to his legs and move them step by step for him. Nor would it be wise to prevent the child from walking for fear that he might injure himself. When we fall ill, we each have an opportunity to grow into a fuller human being as the vital force learns to overcome illness.

Many homeopaths find that children who have had fewer or no vaccinations are on the whole able to overcome acute illnesses more easily than their fully vaccinated counterparts. Though it would be convenient for homeopaths and parents alike, taking a hard-line position on all vaccines for all of the population does not serve children well. Parents must ultimately decide for themselves whether or not they think the risks of each vaccine outweigh the benefits. Many factors will inform that decision: family history, age and strength of the child, likeliness of exposure to each disease, lifestyle, personal beliefs, advice from family health care providers, and books and information. All that could be said in defense of both sides of this issue would require volumes to do it justice. Parents are encouraged to explore the many books and articles written on this topic before vaccinating their child. See "Suggested Readings" and "Online Book Sources" in the Appendix. Becoming well informed will help you make the decisions you can live with.

Note that homeopathic remedies can be highly effective in treating the diseases most vaccines are meant to protect against, and that some can be administered beforehand as a kind of homeopathic vaccine or prophylaxis, prior to entering circumstances of higher risk. Consult a qualified homeopath for further advice about homeopathic vaccines.

BED-WETTING

Bed-wetting is a common problem and should be considered a normal occurrence until the age of six or seven. Nighttime control of the bladder is usually the last hurdle to be overcome in the toilet training process. Some children take more time than others to complete this developmental step. Often with time and patience it will resolve on its own. Stress and emotional factors—insecurities or fears, the appearance of a new sibling, or family or school difficulties—can play a role. Bed-wetting can also be hereditary. Less often there is a physiological problem; if causative factors are not obvious, you may wish to ask your family doctor about tests to rule out organic causes. Homeopathy can be effective in helping a child overcome bed-wetting. The following remedies are known to help, though constitutional treatment may be necessary.

CAUSTICUM

- Occurs soon after falling asleep or during the first part of the night

- Child sometimes wets his or her pants during the day from laughing, coughing, or sneezing

- Child may have various fears: that something bad will happen or of the dark

- May be worse in winter or during changes in weather; better in summer

EQUISETUM

- For no apparent reason; when no other obvious symptoms are present

- If other remedies have been tried and did not help

KREOSOTE

- Sudden urge to urinate, not enough time to run to the bathroom

- Occurs during the first part of the night

- Child may have dreams of urinating while wetting the bed

- Child is a very sound sleeper, difficult to waken

PULSATILLA

- Sensitive, sweet, gentle, and affectionate child who weeps easily

- Child sleeps on back with hands above head or across abdomen

- Bed-wetting more likely when the room is warm and stuffy; desire for fresh air

SEPIA

- Occurs during the first part of the night

- More often a remedy for girls

- Child loves dancing and vigorous motion

- Child is less expressive emotionally or socially; may prefer to be alone

SULPHUR

- Child with *Sulphur* general characteristics (see Part 6)

- Warm-blooded child who sleeps with feet sticking out of the covers

- Child may have vivid dreams

COMMONSENSE MEASURES

- Limit the amount your child drinks in the evening.

- Take your child to the toilet just before bed.

- If you know the time during the night when your child usually wets, carry him or her to the toilet near that hour and whisper a few words of encouragement. This approach can work well but is less suitable for children who tend to fuss and struggle when awakened during the night, or who stay very much asleep while sitting on the toilet.

- Keep your child well covered at night, especially from the waist down. Getting a chill can promote bed-wetting. If your child tends to kick the covers off, make sure he or she wears warm pajamas.

- More consistency and regularity in the daily routine can provide a greater sense of security and assurance.

- Have patience, and do not reprimand or show disapproval. Your child already knows what is expected and wants to please you. Keep a positive attitude and your child will overcome the problem more easily.

CHICKEN POX

Symptoms commonly appear from ten to twenty-one days after exposure to the chicken pox virus. The first signs are general malaise, fever, with perhaps a headache or sore throat. Next comes a spotty rash, which turns into crops of small water-filled blisters. Over several days to several weeks, these vesicles will erupt, burst, and become crusted over. The virus is contagious from several days before the first symptoms appear until all the vesicles are crusted over. During the various phases of the illness, different remedies may be needed.

ACONITE

- During the initial fever stage

- Sudden onset of fever, with anxiety and restlessness; increased thirst

- Dry cough may be present

ANTIMONIUM CRUDUM

- Very irritable child who wants to be left alone

- Tongue thickly coated white

- Itching of spots worse after bathing or from heat of bed

- Cough or bronchitis may be present

ANTIMONIUM TARTARICUM

- Weak and drowsy

- Wet-sounding cough or bronchitis, with nausea

- Eruptions filled with pus (not clear fluid)

- Rash progressing slowly

BELLADONNA

- During the initial fever stage

- Sudden onset of fever; flushed face; bursting headache; dry, hot skin

- Drowsiness; red, glazed eyes

PULSATILLA

- Child is clingy, weepy, and feels better from sympathy

- Itching worse at night and from warmth; better from open air

- Little or no thirst, even when fever is present

RHUS TOXICODENDRON

- The most common remedy for chicken pox

- Intense itching that is worse at night, when resting, and from scratching

- Much restlessness from itching, causing great difficulty sleeping

SULPHUR

- In the final stage, when needed to resolve prolonged or lingering symptoms

- Much itching, worse from warmth of bed or after a warm bath

COMMONSENSE MEASURES

- Bed rest is not necessary, but quiet activity at home is best.

- Keep the diet light and simple.

- An oatmeal powder added to the bath can help reduce itching. Do not use oatmeal soaps.

- Once the eruptions have begun to crust over, apply *Calendula* spray. This will help to heal them quickly and minimize scarring. Leave it on for a minute or two and gently pat dry. For dry, itchy scabs, follow with *Calendula* ointment.

SEEK PROFESSIONAL HELP

- If cough or other symptoms are severe

- If nothing is helping and you are worried

CIRCUMCISION

Homeopathy can provide safe and gentle relief from the discomfort or bleeding that can accompany circumcision. Often one or two doses is all that is needed.

ARNICA MONTANA

- Give one or two doses before the procedure, and once again right afterward to minimize shock.

STAPHYSAGRIA

- Give one dose after the procedure, about one hour following *Arnica* if pain is evident.

COLIC

Colic is the term for severe abdominal pain that comes and goes sporadically. It is common in babies, especially during the first three months of life, when the digestive tract is still maturing. Most often after three months, colic resolves by itself.

Colic is characterized by painful spasms in the intestines, distension, gas, and often prolonged and distressing crying. Homeopathy can be very effective in treating colic, and many new parents have been won over by homeopathy after giving a remedy to their colicky infant. Often the correct homeopathic medicine will quiet a screaming child within minutes or seconds.

AETHUSA

- Colic from milk intolerance, vomiting of large curds within an hour after feeding

- Severe, projectile vomiting may occur; diarrhea is common

- Baby is typically sweaty, weak, restless, crying

BELLADONNA

- Severe spasms that come and go quickly, causing sudden shrieks

- Baby may arch the back forward or backward

- Abdomen usually hot to the touch

CHAMOMILLA

- A primary colic remedy; extreme irritability, anger, sensitivity to pain

- Must be carried, nothing else satisfies the baby; inconsolable

- Irritable, angry-sounding crying if parents try to put baby down; kicks, screams, arches backward

- Often accompanies teething and/or diarrhea; stools may be green like chopped spinach

COLOCYNTHIS

- Pain better from bending double or drawing knees up

- Better from leaning against something hard, as in pressing belly against the parent's shoulder while being carried or simply lying on stomach

- Much restlessness from pain; thrashing, writhing, or rolling about

DIOSCOREA VILLOSA

- Baby wants to stretch or arch backward to relieve pain

- Pain worse from bending forward

LYCOPODIUM

- Much gas, distension, and rumbling after feeding

- Pain worse from any pressure on abdomen; baby may frown or have a furrowed brow

- Gas pains in breast-feeding baby after the mother eats cabbage, cauliflower, onions, oysters, beans, or peas

- Symptoms worse from 4:00 to 8:00 P.M., or baby may wake with colic around 4:00 A.M.

MAGNESIA PHOSPHORICA

- Likes to lie with knees drawn up, as with *Colocynthis*

- Severe cramping pains, alleviated by very warm applications, such as a hot water bottle

- Better from warm drinks and rubbing

NUX VOMICA

- Very irritable baby who frequently strains to move bowels but cannot

- Painful retching and ineffective attempts to vomit

- Colic in a breast-feeding baby after the mother ingests rich or spicy food, alcohol, or drugs

PULSATILLA

- Colic in a breast-feeding baby after the mother eats rich or fatty foods

- Baby is sweet and mild in temperament and wants affection all the time

- Much pitiful weeping, evoking sympathy more often than children who need *Chamomilla* or *Nux vomica*

COMMONSENSE MEASURES

- Dietary considerations: Breast-feeding mothers should try to avoid eating foods known to cause intestinal gas: brussels sprouts, cabbage, cauliflower, garlic, legumes, and onions; these can contribute to colic in babies. Caffeine, dairy products, chocolate, and sugar may also affect the digestibility of mothers' milk. Often foods that give a mother gas will affect her baby similarly. Sometimes switching to formula feeding or introducing solid foods can stress a baby's digestive system. In other instances the diet of the mother or child has little or no influence over the colic. Fortunately, a remedy can help without needing to pin-point the cause. When the cause is known, however, every effort should be made to remove it.

- Tension during feeding time can affect the baby's digestion. Find a relaxing place to nurse where you can both feel comfortable. Make sure the baby isn't gulping down air while nursing. If you feel your baby isn't feeding properly, contact your health care provider, pediatrician, or a lactation consultant.

- Fennel tea or chamomile tea is often helpful to babies with colic. For fennel tea, simmer 1 teaspoon of fennel seed for ten minutes in 1 pint of water. Strain and give warm or tepid. Chamomile tea should be steeped for one minute only, then strained. Give tea with an eyedropper or spoon, or from a bottle.

SEEK PROFESSIONAL HELP
- If colic is severe and/or persistent

CONJUNCTIVITIS (PINKEYE) AND STIES

CONJUNCTIVITIS

Often symptoms of conjunctivitis, or pinkeye, start in one eye and spread to the other. Common symptoms of this infection include itching, burning, redness, swelling, pain, tearing, and sticky discharge from the eye. Select from among the following remedies for relief.

APIS MELLIFICA
- Itching, stinging, and burning with profuse hot tears

- Marked swelling of eyelid

- Worse from warmth; better from cool applications

- Very sensitive to touch; may feel like there is sand in eye

ARGENTUM NITRICUM

- Eyelids swollen and red

- Thick, creamy discharge from eye

- Better from cool applications

- Sensitivity to light

ARSENICUM ALBUM

- Burning pain, better from warm applications

- Discharge or tears are acrid and burning

- Anxiety and restlessness

BELLADONNA

- Inflammation with sudden onset

- Very bloodshot eyes

- Sensitivity to light

EUPHRASIA

- Red, inflamed eyes with profuse burning tears

- Tears irritate and redden skin

- Pain as of sand or grit in eye

FERRUM PHOSPHORICUM

- Early stage of onset, with few distinguishing symptoms

HEPAR SULPHURIS

- Advanced inflammation, with thick discharge

- Extreme sensitivity to pain, worse from touch and cold air

MERCURIUS VIVUS

- Yellow-green burning discharge; advanced inflammation

- Worse from heat and during the night

- Eruptions or crusts around eyes

PULSATILLA

- Thick, bland, yellow, green, or whitish discharge

- Much itching and burning at night

- Eyelids glued together upon waking

- Better from cool applications

COMMONSENSE MEASURES

- Avoid touching or rubbing the eyes to prevent recontamination or spreading of the infection to the other eye or other people. If you do touch the eye, wash your hands promptly and thoroughly. Since conjunctivitis is highly contagious, children should be kept home from school until the condition has cleared.

- Bathing the eye can be very soothing and washes away mucus and debris. Add 4 drops of *Euphrasia* mother tincture to 2 ounces of distilled water or sterile saline solution. Use a clean eyedropper to flush the eye with the solution, taking care not to touch the tip of the dropper to the eye. Repeat three or four times per day. When there is marked pus, discharge, or crust, a *Hypericum* and *Calendula* lotion is preferred: Add 2 drops of each mother tincture to 2 ounces of distilled water or sterile saline solution. Bathe affected eye as just described, and gently wipe the outside with a clean cloth dipped in the lotion.

SEEK PROFESSIONAL HELP

- If there is any loss of vision

- If pain, redness, swelling, or discharge is severe

- If pupils are irregular in size or shape

- If bright light causes much pain

STIES

An infected pimple or boil on the margin of the eyelid, a sty can be quite painful. Typically the spot becomes red and inflamed, and fills with pus. Eventually the sty will burst and heal. A homeopathic remedy can aid the healing process and bring considerable pain relief. Children with recurrent sties will benefit from constitutional treatment.

APIS MELLIFICA

- Markedly swollen eyelid, with burning and stinging pain

- Better from cool compress; worse from any warmth

BELLADONNA

- Sty appears very quickly with much redness

- Sensitivity to light with dilated pupils

HEPAR SULPHURIS

- Very painful and sensitive to touch and cold air

- Sty comes to a head very slowly

- Better from a warm compress

LYCOPODIUM

- Sties on right eye, often on inner corner of eyelid

PULSATILLA

- Primary remedy when there are few other symptoms

- Especially occurring on upper lid

- Yellow-green discharge may be present

STAPHYSAGRIA

- Tendency to recurrent sties, with itching

- May be caused by suppressed anger or upset after an argument

- Tends to form a hard lump

SULPHUR

- Very hot, red, and burning sties

- Worse from heat and bathing

COMMONSENSE MEASURES

- Bathe the eye several times a day with water as hot as is tolerable. This will help soften the sty and bring it to a head.

SEEK PROFESSIONAL HELP

- If vision is impaired

- If symptoms are severe or do not resolve within three days

- If there are accompanying symptoms of illness, such as fever or weakness

CROUP

Croup is a type of cough caused by an irritation of the larynx; it sounds harsh, hoarse, and barking. Croup occurs most often in children aged three months to four years. Homeopathic remedies are often very effective in helping shorten the course of the illness. The first three remedies are often indicated during onset. More information about these remedies can be found in "Colds, Coughs, and Bronchitis." The last three remedies are best suited to more developed cases.

ACONITE

- Primary remedy for croup that comes on suddenly at night

- Sudden onset of dry cough after exposure to cold, dry weather

- Hoarse, barking cough with restlessness, anxiety, and fear

BELLADONNA

- Sudden high fever with dry, painful cough

- Face is flushed red, hot and dry; eyes may be glazed or pupils dilated

FERRUM PHOSPHORICUM

- Early stages of dry cough

- Fever, flushed cheeks

- No other distinguishing symptoms

Aconite, Belladonna, and *Ferrum phosphoricum* may be given every thirty minutes to one hour during the first signs of the cough if symptoms are strong. Two or three doses should quiet the cough either for a while or completely. The following three remedies should be considered after the first twenty-four hours.

DROSERA

- Violent episodes of ringing or barking cough

- Cough immediately worse on lying down at night

- Coughing fits with difficulty catching breath; fits may end in vomiting

- Worse from eating and especially from drinking

HEPAR SULPHURIS
- Useful in advanced, later stages

- Wet, rattling mucus with cough; loose cough, worse in the morning

- Very chilly and sensitive to anything cold: food, drinks, air

- Exposure to cold air brings on coughing and sneezing

- Child is often anxious, quite irritable, and prone to angry outbursts

- *Hepar sulphuris* is often given after *Spongia* when indicated

SPONGIA TOSTA
- Primary remedy for croup

- Hoarse, dry, ringing, or barking cough; often worse around midnight

- Cough resembles a seal's bark or the sound of a saw going through wood

- Cough from a tickle in throat, better from warm foods and drinks

- *Spongia* is often given after *Aconite* when indicated

COMMONSENSE MEASURES
- Steam inhalation is often extremely helpful.

- See "Coughs, Colds, and Bronchitis" for general home care measures.

DIAPER RASH

Some babies and children are more prone to diaper rashes than others. Homeopathic remedies can be very helpful in soothing and healing a sore bottom. If diaper rash is severe or recurs frequently, constitutional homeopathic treatment is recommended.

CALENDULA

- *Calendula* is a wonderfully soothing remedy for diaper rash and may be applied as an ointment, gel, spray, oil, or a powder. The spray, gel, and powder have the advantage of allowing the skin to breathe, but the ointment provides a good barrier against urine and feces, which can irritate. The best strategy is to allow the skin to breathe as much as possible during the day, reserving the use of ointment for when the baby is likely to remain wet or soiled for a period of time, such as nighttime or during naps. The oil mixed with a little warm water makes an excellent solution for routine cleaning of the baby's bottom.

COMMONSENSE MEASURES

- Change diapers promptly when wet or soiled.

- Expose the baby's bottom to fresh air and sunshine as often as possible.

- Be sure your laundry soap is nonirritating.

EARACHE

Childhood earaches are very common occurrences. Although doctors often prescribe antibiotics for ear infections, many current studies cast doubt not only on their effectiveness but also on their appropriateness in many situations. Many children are given antibiotics for

ear pain where no bacterial infection exists. But such overprescrip-
tion of antibiotics has far-reaching consequences. "Losing the Battle
of the Bugs," a cover story in *U.S. News & World Report* in May 1999,
stated, "The rampant inappropriate use of [antibiotics] for colds and
other ailments is contributing to the rise of resistant bacterial strains
that cannot be treated. As many as half of outpatient antibiotic pre-
scriptions a year are written unnecessarily, according to the Federal
Centers for Disease Control and Prevention."

Many parents today are discovering safer and more effective means
of treating ear infections. Homeopathy provides a way of curing an
infection while strengthening the resistance to it, whether it is bacterial or viral. The most common type of earache is middle ear infection, or otitis media. Both acute and chronic ear complaints can be
successfully treated with homeopathy. Chronic or frequently recurring ear infections are best handled with constitutional treatment.

The following three remedies are often most helpful during the
early onset of ear pain. When the remedy is chosen well and given
soon enough, progress of the infection may be stopped altogether.

ACONITE

- Sudden onset of ear pain with restlessness, anxiety, and fear

- After exposure to cold, dry wind

- Pain comes on at night or is worse at night with fever and thirst

- External ear is hot and painful, may be red; face often flushed

BELLADONNA

- Sudden onset of ear pain, often right-sided, less often left-sided

- Face is bright red, hot, and dry, with fever but no thirst

- Child may be irritable, with glassy eyes and dilated pupils

- Ear looks very red; pain is throbbing or piercing

FERRUM PHOSPHORICUM

- Early stage of ear pain, onset is not forceful

- Flushed cheeks

- No other distinguishing characteristics

The following group of remedies is suited to a variety of other types of earaches.

CHAMOMILLA

- Extremely painful earache, great sensitivity to pain; strong aversion to being touched

- Unbearably irritable from pain; demanding, yet nothing pleases child

- Angry-sounding crying and screaming

- Must be carried, protests vehemently if put down

- One cheek red and hot, the other pale and cool

HEPAR SULPHURIS

- Very sensitive to pain, irritable, and shrieking from pain; worse from touch and at night

- Very chilly and sensitive to anything cold: air, wind, drafts, drinks, food

- Better from wrapping ear, from keeping warm in general

- Sensation of a splinter in ear, offensive smelling discharge from ear

LYCOPODIUM

- Right-sided infection, or begins on right and spreads to left

- Worse between 4:00 and 8:00 P.M.

- Worse from cold air or drafts

- Ear feels stopped up; buzzing or ringing in affected ear

___

MERCURIUS VIVUS

- Ear pain with swollen glands and sore throat; worse at night

- Pain may extend to face and teeth

- Offensive smelling discharge from ear

- Sweaty, increased saliva, foul breath

___

PULSATILLA

- Begins with a common cold that progresses into ear infection

- Much pitiful crying from pain; clingy, wants to be held and caressed

- Ear feels stopped up, with pulsating or bursting sensation

- Worse at night, in a warm, closed room

- Better in open air and from being rocked or carried gently

- Usually thirstless; bland discharge from ear

COMMONSENSE MEASURES

- Put a few drops of warmed *Mullein* oil (*verbascum*) in the affected ear every three or four hours, but only if there is no discharge from the ear. Have the child lie on his or her side for five minutes or more, so the oil slides all the way in.

- A warm carrot or onion compress can also give welcome relief from ear pain. Warm a slice of onion, wrap it in a handkerchief, and lay it gently against the ear. Put a woolen ski cap or similar hat on the head to cover the ears. This holds the compress in place and helps retain heat. With a carrot, grate it and heat briefly in a pan. Then place it in the center of a handkerchief and tie it off to make a compressible, ear-size ball. Apply in the same manner as the onion. A chamomile compress can be made in a similar manner.

SEEK PROFESSIONAL HELP

- If significant pain persists for more than twenty-four hours

- If the bony area behind the ear becomes painful, red, or swollen

- If the child has a stiff neck with high fever, drowsiness, and headache

GROWING PAINS

Sometimes during a growth spurt, or for no apparent reason at all, children experience pains in their legs. Growing pains usually occur in children between ages six and thirteen, and are most commonly experienced at night. Give one of the following if indicated, in a 6C potency, three times daily for up to two weeks. Discontinue when there is improvement, and repeat only as needed.

CALCAREA PHOSPHORICA

- Primary remedy for aching in legs caused by very rapid growth

- Legs feel restless, sometimes with a tingling or crawling sensation

GUAIACUM

- Worse in cold, damp weather and from exertion

- Often worse in thighs

- Better from cool applications and applying local pressure

PHOSPHORIC ACID

- Tearing pains in legs, as though the bones were being scraped

- General tiredness after a period of prolonged stress

- Child may stumble easily and make missteps

NOSEBLEEDS

Nosebleeds are common occurrences, and some children are more susceptible than others. Whether the nosebleed is caused by an injury to the nose, a fall, a foreign object, or from blowing or picking the nose, a homeopathic remedy can help stop bleeding. In children who tend to get repeated nosebleeds, constitutional treatment may be needed. For nosebleeds that accompany acute illnesses, refer to other relevant sections of this book. You may also wish to refer to "Bleeding" for additional remedies.

ACONITE

- When great anxiety, restlessness, or fear are present

- Bright red blood

- Numbness in nose may accompany bleeding

ARNICA MONTANA

- Primary remedy for nosebleed from an injury, blow, or fall

PHOSPHORUS

- Nosebleed with bright red blood; may be difficult to stop bleeding

- From forceful nose blowing

- If *Arnica* has not stopped the bleeding

COMMONSENSE MEASURES

- Apply pressure: Gently but firmly pinch the middle of the bridge of the nose for five to ten minutes until bleeding stops. Apply ice as well if bleeding is persistent, or if swelling and bruising are anticipated (in an injury).

SEEK PROFESSIONAL HELP

- If the preceding measures do not help

- If nosebleeds are a recurrent problem

TEETHING

Teething problems are not uncommon in children. At approximately six months of age the first "milk teeth" appear, and usually by the time a child is two and a half, he or she will have grown in all twenty baby teeth. Along the way, discomforts may occur. Common symptoms include: pain in the immediate gum and tooth area, drooling, loose stools, and fever, all of which may be accompanied by whining, crying, restlessness, or irritability. When the distress is due to slow or delayed teething, homeopathy can be very effective in stimulating the eruption of teeth while alleviating attending discomforts.

ACONITE

- Severe pain accompanied by great restlessness and anxiety

- Inflamed gums, fever may be present

- Worse from cold drinks and cold air

BELLADONNA

- Severe pain causing child to kick, scream, or bite

- Cheeks, lips, and gums may be quite red, with or without fever

CALCAREA CARBONICA

- Slow or delayed teething

- Late developmental features: closure of fontanelles, sitting, crawling, or walking

- Puts fingers in mouth

- Often seen in plump, fair-haired, large-headed children

- Perspiration of the head; sour odor of sweat, stools, and vomit

- Constipation or diarrhea

CALCAREA PHOSPHORICA

- Slow or delayed development with late closure of fontanelles, late walking, etc.

- Perspiration of head

- Often thin or emaciated

- Peevish, irritable, whiny; desires to be carried

- Diarrhea with marked flatulence

CHAMOMILLA

- Primary teething remedy unless another is clearly indicated

- Extreme irritability, anger, sensitivity to pain; child may strike or kick

- Great impatience; demands things then refuses them when offered

- Inconsolable, nothing pleases

- Must be carried, cries angrily when put down

- One cheek hot and red, the other cheek pale

- Diarrhea with green stools like chopped spinach

KREOSOTE

- Very inflamed, spongy gums; bleed easily

- Great pain with irritability, restlessness; nothing pleases

- Rapid decay of teeth as soon as they appear

- Offensive breath

COMMONSENSE MEASURES

- Give your baby something to chew on, preferably something cold. A frozen biscuit, bagel, or an ice cube wrapped in a frozen washcloth can be a great comfort. Sometimes a favorite toy will have just the right feel in the mouth.

SEEK PROFESSIONAL HELP

- If the preceding recommendations do not help

THRUSH

Thrush is an overgrowth of yeast that occurs in the mouth and appears as white patches in the mouth and/or on the tongue. Sometimes the tissues of the mouth may swell, and there can be considerable pain and distress when eating, drinking, or sucking. Homeopathy can be highly effective in treating oral thrush.

BORAX

- A primary remedy for thrush and mouth ulcers

- White spots and patches, much pain when sucking, eating

- Mouth feels hot to the mother's nipple

- Marked fear of downward motion

HYDRASTIS

- When thrush appears more yellow

- Tongue streaked yellow; yellow mucus

KALI MURIATICUM

- When no other clear symptoms are present

- Most helpful at onset

- Tongue may have grayish coating at base; patchy tongue

MERCURIUS VIVUS

- Offensive breath and excessive salivation; may drool all over pillow

- Sores and ulcers in mouth

COMMONSENSE MEASURES

- Gargle with a solution of *Calendula* tincture and water: 20 drops tincture to 4 ounces warm water. Goldenseal tincture (*Hydrastis*) is also excellent for this purpose and may be used instead or split with the *Calendula* (10 drops each). Goldenseal is extremely bitter, though, and many children dislike it. If gargling is not possible, gently wipe inside of mouth with the solution using sterile gauze or a cotton swab.

SEEK PROFESSIONAL HELP

- If the condition is severely painful or recurrent

WORMS

Pinworms infest the rectum and can cause itching at the anus, colicky abdominal pains, and increased irritability. A child can easily reintroduce the infestation by way of fingers in the mouth after scratching the itchy bottom. Worms are also easily transmitted to other family members.

CINA

- The primary remedy for pinworms

- Itching anus, with increased hunger and irritability

- Nose picking and teeth grinding; dark circles under eyes

TEUCRIUM

- Itching anus and nose, worse in the evening

- Restless sleep

- Complains of a crawling sensation in rectum after bowel movements

COMMONSENSE MEASURES

- Careful attention to hygiene is a must. Wash the hands properly after every bathroom use.

- Eliminate sugar from the diet as much as possible. Worms thrive on it.

- Eating pumpkin seeds and *pepitas* (their green variety) can help eliminate worms.

- Put Hypercal ointment in the anal area to soothe it and to discourage the worms' mobility.

- Watch for signs of infestation in other household members and treat accordingly.

SEEK PROFESSIONAL HELP

- If worms are a recurrent problem for the child or family

- If there is no improvement within four or five days

PART 6

MATERIA MEDICA:

DESCRIPTIONS OF THE MAJOR REMEDIES

Use the following descriptions for quick reference when selecting a remedy for a particular ailment. These show a broad range of symptoms that each remedy can cure but many finer details are not listed here. For a more in-depth knowledge of these remedies and more, see "Suggested Readings."

ACONITE
(Monkshood)

COMMON AILMENTS
- First stages of fever or acute inflammation
- Earache, sore throat, respiratory infection
- Emotional shock with fear of death
- Eye injury

CHARACTERISTIC SYMPTOMS
- Ailments that come on suddenly after exposure to cold or wind
- Ailments after a shock or accident with fear, panic, and anxiety
- Acute illnesses, which come on suddenly in the middle of the night
- Specific for shock after witnessing a horrible accident, natural disaster, or other disturbing event

- Thirsty

- Hot, may have one cheek red, the other pale

___

MENTAL AND EMOTIONAL SYMPTOMS

- Sudden fear and anxiety in a person who is usually strong and vital

- Person may fear he or she is going to die and even predict the time of death

- Panic attacks

- Restlessness

___

WORSE FROM

- Dry wind, cold, night, lying on the affected side

___

BETTER FROM

- Fresh air, rest

ALLIUM CEPA
(Red onion)

___

COMMON AILMENTS

- Hay fever

- Common cold

___

CHARACTERISTIC SYMPTOMS

- Acrid, burning discharges

- Bland tearing of eyes

- Desire for raw onions

MENTAL AND EMOTIONAL SYMPTOMS
- Dullness

WORSE FROM
- Warmth

- Damp

- Evening

BETTER FROM
- Cool air

- Bathing

ANTIMONIUM TARTARICUM
(Tartar emetic)

COMMON AILMENTS
- Respiratory infections and complaints

CHARACTERISTIC SYMPTOMS
- Rattling and fullness in chest

- Little expectoration of mucus

- Desire for acidic foods or apples

- Tongue coated white

- Weakness

MENTAL AND EMOTIONAL SYMPTOMS
- Doesn't want to be looked at

- Apathetic, dull, or drowsy

WORSE FROM

- Heat

- Warm rooms

- Lying down

- Overeating

- Changes of weather

BETTER FROM

- Spitting up mucus

- Sitting up

- Moving around

- Cold air

APIS MELLIFICA
(Honeybee)

COMMON AILMENTS

- Allergies

- Bites

- Hives

- Cystitis

- Sore throat

CHARACTERISTIC SYMPTOMS

- Burning and stinging pains

- Hot and swollen

- Thirstless

MENTAL AND EMOTIONAL SYMPTOMS

- Fruitlessly busy, like a busy bee

- Anger and/or jealousy

- Clumsiness

WORSE FROM

- Heat

- Touch

- Pressure

- Late afternoon

BETTER FROM

- Cold—applications, bathing, air

- Movement

ARNICA MONTANA
(Mountain daisy or leopard's bane)

COMMON AILMENTS

- Injuries and trauma

- Surgery (before and after)

- Jet lag

CHARACTERISTIC SYMPTOMS

- Soreness and bruised feeling

- Tendency to bruising and passive bleeding following injury

- Muscle ache from straining or overexertion (e.g., gardening, exercise)

MENTAL AND EMOTIONAL SYMPTOMS

- Says "I'm all right" when clearly injured

- Fear or aversion to being touched

WORSE FROM

- Touch

- Cold

- Movement

BETTER FROM

- Lying with head low

- Fresh air

- Cold bath

- Sitting up

ARSENICUM ALBUM
(White arsenic)

COMMON AILMENTS

- Gastrointestinal complaints

- Food poisoning

- Cold and flu

- Diarrhea of travelers

CHARACTERISTIC SYMPTOMS

- Burning pains alleviated by heat

- Desire for company

- Restlessness, anxiety, and chilliness

- Thirst for small sips

- Acrid discharges

MENTAL AND EMOTIONAL SYMPTOMS

- Anxiety driving the person from room to room

- Fearful, may even fear dying from the illness

- Neat and tidy (would never leave dirty tissues lying around)

- Does not want to be left alone out of fear

WORSE FROM

- Night, especially after midnight

- Cold food and drinks

- Spoiled meat, fruit, or other foods

- Any exertion

BETTER FROM

- Warmth—food, applications, wrapping

- Movement—shifting position

- Having head elevated

BELLADONNA
(Deadly nightshade)

COMMON AILMENTS

- Fever

- Cold, cough, flu

- Ear infection

- Headache

- Teething problems

- Sore throat/swollen glands

- Sunstroke

CHARACTERISTIC SYMPTOMS
- Suddenness and violence of symptoms

- Ailments from being chilled or overheated

- Heat, throbbing, redness

- Pupils dilated; eyes glassy

- Dryness

- Desire for lemons or lemonade

- Delirium or hallucination with fever

MENTAL AND EMOTIONAL SYMPTOMS
- In children: "an angel when well, a devil when sick" and may be very angry; may strike, bite, or kick

- Frightening hallucinations during fevers

WORSE FROM
- Heat, the sun

- 3:00 P.M. (a common time for the onset of a *Belladonna* illness)

- Drafts

- Having the hair cut

BETTER FROM

- Light covering; cool applications

- Resting in darkness

- Bending backward

BRYONIA ALBA
(Wild hops)

COMMON AILMENTS

- Influenza

- Respiratory infections

- Headache

- Back or other musculoskeletal pain

- Digestive complaints

- Constipation

CHARACTERISTIC SYMPTOMS

- Dryness of all mucous membranes

- Any movement hurts

- Stitching pains

- Thirst for large quantities of cold water at intervals

MENTAL AND EMOTIONAL SYMPTOMS

- Irritable and grumpy; "the bear"

- Wants to be left alone

- Wants to go home (even if home already)

- Preoccupation with or talk of business

___
WORSE FROM
- Any movement (even breathing in chest ailments)

- Hot weather

___
BETTER FROM
- Sustained pressure on painful part

- Cool air

CALCAREA CARBONICA
(Calcium carbonate)

___
COMMON AILMENTS
- Cold

- Glandular swelling

- Sore throat

- Menstrual problems

- Teething

___
CHARACTERISTIC SYMPTOMS
- Chilly but easily overheated

- Sweat on head and neck

- Sour-smelling sweat

- Difficult teething

- Very susceptible to colds

- Desire for sweets and soft-boiled eggs

- Ailments from exertion and overwork

- Often overweight

MENTAL AND EMOTIONAL SYMPTOMS

- Many fears and anxieties caused by worry about security

- Overwhelmed with responsibility; carries the world on his or her shoulders

- Fear of heights, airplanes, earthquakes

- Fear of animals: dogs, mice, insects, and spiders

- May be slow and plodding, phlegmatic; stubborn

- Methodical, hardworking, and responsible

WORSE FROM

- Cold

- Change of weather

- Pressure of clothing

- Not eating

- Exertion, climbing stairs

- Before menstrual period

- Sleeping

- Getting wet

BETTER FROM

- Dry weather

- Morning

- Rubbing

- Lying on back

CARBO VEGETABILIS
(Vegetable charcoal)

COMMON AILMENTS

- Respiratory ailments

- Whooping cough

- Shock, collapse, fainting

- Stomach complaints and flatulence

CHARACTERISTIC SYMPTOMS

- Very sluggish, no vitality

- Cold

- Needs to be fanned

- Cold extremities

- Blue extremities

- Gassy

- Aversion to tight clothing around waist

- Ailments after a debilitating illness

MENTAL AND EMOTIONAL SYMPTOMS

- Indifference and listlessness

- Fear of dark

WORSE FROM

- Warmth

- Loss of body fluids

- Overeating

BETTER FROM

- Belching and passing gas

- Cool air, especially a fan

- Putting feet up or lying down

CHAMOMILLA
(German chamomile)

COMMON AILMENTS

- Teething

- Ear infection

- Diarrhea

- Colic

- Fever

- Childbirth

CHARACTERISTIC SYMPTOMS

- Extreme oversensitivity to pain

- Unbearable pain

- Wants to be carried

- Desires something, then rejects it

- One cheek red, the other pale (in teething infants)

- Cries out in sleep from pain

- Ailments after drinking coffee

MENTAL AND EMOTIONAL SYMPTOMS
- Extremely irritable, ugly, and angry from pain

- Child cries when put down, kicks and screams

- Doesn't want to be spoken to or touched (except to be carried)

WORSE FROM
- Anger

- Night

- Teething

- Cold

- Coffee

BETTER FROM
- Being carried

- Sweating

- Rocking

COCCULUS INDICA
(Indian cockle)

COMMON AILMENTS
- Motion sickness

- Vertigo

- Jet lag

- Ailments after loss of sleep

- Morning sickness

CHARACTERISTIC SYMPTOMS

- Ailments from stress

- Reactions slowed down

- Nausea from seeing or smelling food

- Aversion to open air

- Salivation and extreme thirst

MENTAL AND EMOTIONAL SYMPTOMS

- Takes a long time to answer

- Doesn't want to be disturbed or interrupted

- Worried

- Feeling that everything is slowed down

- Oversensitive

WORSE FROM

- Motion

- Minor irritations

- Loss of sleep

- Thinking of or smelling food

BETTER FROM

- Lying down

- Warmth

COFFEA CRUDA
(Coffee)

COMMON AILMENTS
- Insomnia

- Overstimulation and excitement

- Toothache

CHARACTERISTIC SYMPTOMS
- Overactivity of mind

- Rushing thoughts

- Oversensitivity to pain

- Quick action

- Aversion to open air though hot

- Acute senses, especially hearing

- Sleeplessness

MENTAL AND EMOTIONAL SYMPTOMS
- See "Characteristic Symptoms"

WORSE FROM
- Noise

- Touch

- Smell

- Overeating

- Too much joy

- Warm water in mouth

BETTER FROM

- Rest

- Ice water in mouth (toothache)

EUPATORIUM PERFOLIATUM
(Boneset)

COMMON AILMENTS

- Flu

CHARACTERISTIC SYMPTOMS

- Feeling like bones are broken

- Deep aching in bones

- Restlessness not relieved by motion

- Strong desire for cold drinks and ice cream

- Chill in small of back

- No perspiration

MENTAL AND EMOTIONAL SYMPTOMS

- Not marked

WORSE FROM

- Cold air

BETTER FROM

- Perspiration

EUPHRASIA
(Eyebright)

COMMON AILMENTS

- Hay fever

- Eye ailments

CHARACTERISTIC SYMPTOMS

- Burning tears with bland nasal discharge

- Acrid tears irritate and redden eyes and cheeks

- Aversion to light, eyes blink

- Swelling

MENTAL AND EMOTIONAL SYMPTOMS

- Not marked

WORSE FROM

- Sun

- Wind

- Evening

- Being in bed

BETTER FROM

- Open air

- Blinking

- Wiping eyes

FERRUM PHOSPHORICUM
(Iron phosphate)

COMMON AILMENTS
- Early stages of inflammatory illness: colds, cough, flu, sore throat

CHARACTERISTIC SYMPTOMS
- Lack of distinguishing symptoms

- Flushed and hot face (may be just cheeks)

- Deafness after colds

MENTAL AND EMOTIONAL SYMPTOMS
- Anxiety at night

WORSE FROM
- Night

- Motion

BETTER FROM
- Lying down

GELSEMIUM
(Yellow jasmine)

COMMON AILMENTS
- Flu

- Anticipatory anxiety: exam fears, stage fright

- Ailments after hearing bad news

- Headache

CHARACTERISTIC SYMPTOMS

- Complaints come on slowly

- Weakness and lethargy

- Dullness with droopy eyelids and dusky face

- Tongue feels heavy and thick

- Fever without thirst

- Trembling

MENTAL AND EMOTIONAL SYMPTOMS

- Anxiety with apprehension, especially about upcoming ordeals: exams, public speaking

- Difficulty in concentration, dullness or confusion

- Feels grief but cannot cry

WORSE FROM

- Fear and fright

- Emotions

- Humidity

- Spring

- Before a thunderstorm

BETTER FROM

- Profuse urination

- Perspiring

HEPAR SULPHURIS CALCAREUM
(Calcium sulphide)

COMMON AILMENTS

- Sore throat

- Respiratory ailments

- Ear infection

- Boils, abscesses, infected wounds

CHARACTERISTIC SYMPTOMS

- Very chilly—can't get warm

- Extremely oversensitive—to pain, touch, the least little draft

- Craving for vinegar and other acidic foods

- Sticking or stitching pains

- All discharges foul

- Very sweaty but won't uncover

MENTAL AND EMOTIONAL SYMPTOMS

- Extremely irritable, discontented with everything

- Contradictory

- Violent impulses

WORSE FROM

- Cold—air, wind, food, drinks

- Touch

BETTER FROM

- Heat

- Damp

HYPERICUM
(St. John's wort)

COMMON AILMENTS

- Injuries to nerves in head, neck, spine, coccyx

- Crush injuries of fingers and toes

- Penetrating wounds, where pains shoot along nerves

- Ill effects from head or spinal injury: headache, dizziness, seizures, asthma

CHARACTERISTIC SYMPTOMS

- Sharp, shooting pains that run along nerves

- Pains appear suddenly and disappear gradually

MENTAL AND EMOTIONAL SYMPTOMS

- Dullness after head injury

- Mistakes in writing, omits letters

- Mistakes in speaking, uses wrong words

WORSE FROM

- Injury

- Change of weather

- Cold air

BETTER FROM
- Lying quietly

IGNATIA AMARA
(St. Ignatius bean)

COMMON AILMENTS
- Ailments that appear after grief, disappointment, worry, or shocking news

CHARACTERISTIC SYMPTOMS
- Spasmodic symptoms: sighing, sobs, lump in throat, mouth twitching

- Headache with sensation of a nail being driven into side of head

- Symptoms contradict or alternate

- Aversion to fruit

- Aversion to smoke

MENTAL AND EMOTIONAL SYMPTOMS
- Silent grief, with or without anger

- Tearful; hysterical sobbing

- Very sensitive and nervous

- Laughs and cries alternately

- Wants to be alone to cry

- Brooding, self-reproaching, idealistic

WORSE FROM
- Emotions

- Air

- Smells

- Coffee; smoke

- Consolation

BETTER FROM
- Changing position

- Being alone

- Hard pressure

- Lying on the painful side

IPECACUANHA
(Ipecac root)

COMMON AILMENTS
- Nausea and vomiting

- Whooping cough

- Respiratory ailments

- Bleeding

CHARACTERISTIC SYMPTOMS
- Nausea not relieved by vomiting

- Thirstlessness

- Profuse salivation

- Nausea with a clean tongue

- Children vomit with common cold

WORSE FROM
- Warmth

- Overeating

BETTER FROM
- Open air

KALI BICHROMICUM
(Potassium bichromate)

COMMON AILMENTS
- Sinus infection

- Headache

CHARACTERISTIC SYMPTOMS
- Thick, stringy, gluey nasal discharges

- Chilly, but worse in hot weather

- Worse from 2:00 to 3:00 A.M.

- Pains in small spots (patient can point to exact spot)

- Problems recur at the same time each day or season

MENTAL AND EMOTIONAL SYMPTOMS
- Not marked

- May prefer routine, order, and predictability

WORSE FROM

- Cold

- Morning

- 2:00 to 3:00 A.M.

BETTER FROM

- Heat

- Motion

- Eating

- Napping

KALI CARBONICUM
(Potassium carbonate)

COMMON AILMENTS

- Back pain

- Respiratory ailments

CHARACTERISTIC SYMPTOMS

- Stitching pains

- Chilly with lots of sweating

MENTAL AND EMOTIONAL SYMPTOMS

- Feels emotions in stomach

- Strong sense of duty

WORSE FROM

- 2:00 to 4:00 A.M.

- Cold

- Lying on painful part

BETTER FROM
- Warmth

LACHESIS
(Venom of the bushmaster snake)

COMMON AILMENTS
- Sore throat

- Poisonous bites, boils, abscesses

- Headache

- Menstrual and menopausal complaints, PMS

CHARACTERISTIC SYMPTOMS
- Left-sided complaints or left side first, moving to right

- Feels worse after falling asleep or on waking in the morning

- Cannot bear anything constricting—jewelry, clothing (e.g., no turtlenecks), or blankets—especially near the throat

- Oversensitive to heat and oppressive weather

- Purple discoloration of affected areas

MENTAL AND EMOTIONAL SYMPTOMS
- Very talkative; jesting, sarcasm

- Intense, passionate

- Suspiciousness, jealousy, desire for revenge

WORSE FROM

- Sleep

- Hot weather

- Constriction or pressure of clothing or bedclothes

- Heat in any form

- Empty swallowing

- Before menstrual period

BETTER FROM

- Any discharges—especially during menstrual flow

- Open air

- Cold drinks

LEDUM PALUSTRE

(Marsh tea or wild rosemary)

COMMON AILMENTS

- Bites and stings

- Puncture wounds

- Black eye

CHARACTERISTIC SYMPTOMS

- Wound or bite is cold to touch

- Chilly, but heat is intolerable

- Black after injury

WORSE FROM

- Heat

BETTER FROM

- Cold bathing and air

LYCOPODIUM
(Club moss)

COMMON AILMENTS

- Gastric upsets and digestive problems

- Sore throat

- Earache

- Respiratory illnesses

- Impotence

CHARACTERISTIC SYMPTOMS

- Much gas and bloating

- Right-sided complaints or move from right to left

- Desire for sweets

- Anticipation anxiety

- Worse from 4:00 to 8:00 P.M. and 3:00 to 4:00 A.M.

- Desire for warm drinks and food

MENTAL AND EMOTIONAL SYMPTOMS

- Lack of self-confidence and anxiety when undertaking something new

- May project inflated persona to compensate for poor self-confidence

- May be bossy at home but nice to those outside the family

- Feels helpless

- Fear: responsibilities, commitment, failure

- Angry when waking in the morning

WORSE FROM
- Pressure of clothing

- Warmth

- Eating

- 4:00 to 8:00 P.M.

- Waking

BETTER FROM
- Warm food and drinks

- Cold applications

- Motion

- Loosening clothing

MERCURIUS VIVUS
(Quicksilver)

COMMON AILMENTS
- Sore throat

- Diarrhea and digestive upsets

- Earache

- Toothache and abscesses

CHARACTERISTIC SYMPTOMS
- Sweaty with offensive-smelling perspiration

- Sensitivity to both hot and cold, like a mercury thermometer

- Swollen glands

- Profuse salivation and bad breath

- Extreme thirst

MENTAL AND EMOTIONAL SYMPTOMS
- Anxiety and restlessness

- Internal feeling of hurry but slow in actions

- Sadness

- Sensitivity to criticism and contradiction

WORSE FROM
- Night

- Lying on right side

- Heat and cold

BETTER FROM
- After sleeping

NATRUM MURIATICUM
(Sodium chloride or common salt)

COMMON AILMENTS

- Cold

- Cold sores

- Allergies

- Grief

- Digestive disturbances

- Sore throat

- Headache

CHARACTERISTIC SYMPTOMS

- Herpes-type eruptions

- Desire for salt

- Mucus discharges like egg whites

- Bloating and water retention

- May have a "mapped" or patchy tongue

- Dryness and cracked lips

- Very thirsty for water

MENTAL AND EMOTIONAL SYMPTOMS

- Feels sad but is averse to being consoled

- Wants to cry but cannot or cries only when alone

- Full of grief or disappointment

- Dwelling on the past, clinging to old traumas

- Vulnerable; sensitive to music

- Perfectionistic or idealistic; most often introverted

- Children are serious, responsible, and well-behaved, like little adults

WORSE FROM
- 10:00 A.M.

- Eating

- Heat of sun

- Consolation

- Seaside

- Exertion

BETTER FROM
- Hard pressure

- Tight clothing

- Lying down and resting

- Fasting

- May be better by seaside

NUX VOMICA
(Poison nut)

COMMON AILMENTS
- Digestive disturbances

- Cold

- Respiratory ailments

- Flu

- Colic

- Hay fever

- Sore throat

- Hangover

CHARACTERISTIC SYMPTOMS

- Oversensitivity to all stimuli

- Complaints after anger

- Sick after overindulgence

- Very chilly

- Craves stimulants: caffeine, alcohol, spicy foods

- Frequent ineffectual urging: to urinate, move bowels, vomit

- Cramping

MENTAL AND EMOTIONAL SYMPTOMS

- Very irritable and easily angered

- Impatient and impulsive

- Sensitive to everything and everybody

- Bossy, ambitious, high achiever

WORSE FROM

- Cold

- Lying on back

- Motion

- Overindulgence in food, tobacco, alcohol, coffee, drugs

- Dry or fresh air

- Loss of sleep

- Morning

- Uncovering

- Tight clothing

BETTER FROM

- Heat

- Hot drinks

- Lying on side

- Sitting

PHOSPHORUS

COMMON AILMENTS

- Cold

- Cough and respiratory ailments

- Digestive disturbances

- Headache

- Nosebleed

- Sore throat

CHARACTERISTIC SYMPTOMS

- Burning pains and heat sensation

- Very thirsty for cold drinks, especially soda

- Bleeding—bright red blood

- Desire for ice cream, sweets, and salty or spicy foods

- Exhaustion or a surge of energy followed by weakness

MENTAL AND EMOTIONAL SYMPTOMS

- Anxiety and fearfulness, especially at night

- Fear of thunderstorms, ghosts, dogs, dark; fear for others

- Very sympathetic

- Oversensitive

WORSE FROM

- Lying on left side

- The slightest thing (emotion, touch, smell, light)

- Cold

- Warm foods

- Changes in weather

- Lack of rest

BETTER FROM

- Eating

- Sleeping, even catnaps

- Being massaged

- Lying on right side

PULSATILLA
(Windflower)

COMMON AILMENTS

- Earache

- Chicken pox

- Cough

- Cold

- Eye inflammation

- Fever

- Headache

- PMS

- Diarrhea and digestive disturbances

- Sore throat

- Teething and toothache

CHARACTERISTIC SYMPTOMS

- Changeable symptoms

- Desire for open air

- Face easily flushes; blushing

- Bland yellow or yellow-green discharges

- Desire for butter, ice cream, hard-boiled eggs, peanut butter

- Aggravation from fatty and rich foods

- Thirstlessness

MENTAL AND EMOTIONAL SYMPTOMS

- Mild, sweet, and affectionate; often timid and childlike

- Yielding, wants to please

- Clingy—wants consolation and to be held

- Fears heights, dark, narrow places, being alone

- Changeable moods; weeps easily; whiny

- Feels abandoned or forsaken

WORSE FROM

- Eating till full

- Stuffy rooms, stale air

- Being overheated

- Before menstrual period

- Warm foods and drinks

- Rich foods or fats

- Puberty and pregnancy

BETTER FROM

- Fresh air

- Consolation

- Sitting erect

- Crying

- Rubbing

- Cold foods and drinks

RHUS TOXICODENDRON
(Poison ivy)

COMMON AILMENTS
- Strains and sprains

- Stiff neck

- Sore throat

- Poison ivy

- Fever

- Cough

- Chicken pox

- Cold sores and herpes

CHARACTERISTIC SYMPTOMS
- Physical and mental restlessness and stiffness

- Starts out stiff but better from motion

- Ailments from getting damp or cold

- Need to stretch

- Desire for milk

- Metallic taste in mouth

MENTAL AND EMOTIONAL SYMPTOMS
- Restlessness

- Anxiety, especially when confined to bed

- May be superstitious

- May become weepy without knowing why

WORSE FROM
- Cold and wet

- Rising after rest

- After midnight

- Before a storm

- Winter

BETTER FROM
- Motion

- Heat and warm applications

- Massage

- Changing position or stretching

- Lying on a hard surface

SEPIA
(Cuttlefish ink)

COMMON AILMENTS
- PMS

- Constipation

- Cough

- Cystitis

- Headache

- Digestive disturbances

- Depression

- Vaginal dryness; loss of libido in women

CHARACTERISTIC SYMPTOMS

- Dragged-down sensation

- Desire for vinegar and chocolate

- Ailments from getting wet

- Better from vigorous exercise and dancing

- Chilly

- Worse in the late afternoon

- Sweaty from the least exertion

- Left-sided symptoms

MENTAL AND EMOTIONAL SYMPTOMS

- Feels stuck

- Indifference or aversion to people (especially family members)

- Wants to be left alone

- Uncommunicative, flat affect

- Cries when telling symptoms

- Sarcastic, critical, and fault finding, especially toward family

WORSE FROM

- Cold

- Before menstrual period

- During and after eating

- 5:00 P.M.

- Sitting quiet and still

- Before thunderstorms

BETTER FROM

- Vigorous exercise

- Dancing

- Warmth

- Cold drinks

- Keeping busy

- Loosening clothing

- Open air

SILICA

(Flint or silicea)

COMMON AILMENTS

- Sore throat

- Ear infection

- Eye inflammation

- Nail problems

- Headache

- Injuries

- Teething and toothache

- Digestive disturbances

- Splinters

CHARACTERISTIC SYMPTOMS

- Chilly

- Ailments after changes of weather (warm to cold)

- Aversion to meat

- Sweaty

- Swollen glands

- Thirsty

- Low stamina

- Mentally overworked

- Fear of needles

MENTAL AND EMOTIONAL SYMPTOMS

- Shyness and lack of confidence

- Nervousness about undertaking new experiences

- May be delicate or refined

- Obstinate but appears yielding

- Very concerned about image

- Conscientious about small details

WORSE FROM

- Cold air, drafts, bathing

- Noise, light, jarring

- Night

- After vaccination

- Milk

BETTER FROM

- Warmth
- Wrapping
- Urinating

SULPHUR

COMMON AILMENTS
- Cold
- Respiratory ailments
- Diarrhea
- Ear infection
- Eye inflammation
- Fever
- Headache
- Sore throat
- Many skin problems

CHARACTERISTIC SYMPTOMS
- Redness and itching
- Burning pains and heat
- Itching
- Offensive-smelling sweat or other discharges
- Desire for sweets and spicy foods
- Bad taste in mouth

- Swollen glands

- Aversion to eggs or fish

- Aversion to washing, especially in children

MENTAL AND EMOTIONAL SYMPTOMS

- Irritable, angry, or argumentative

- Easily embarrassed

- Slow and sluggish; lazy

- Imaginative and theorizing; full of ideas

- Indifferent to personal appearance; untidy

- Self-centered, conceited, egotistical

WORSE FROM

- Bathing

- Heat

- In bed—may kick covers off

- Wearing wool

- Washing

BETTER FROM

- Open air

- Movement

- Dry, warm weather

- Warm drinks

- Sweating

URTICA URENS
(Stinging nettle)

COMMON AILMENTS
- Bites and stings; itching

- Hives

- Burns

CHARACTERISTIC SYMPTOMS
- Burning and stinging

- Swelling

MENTAL AND EMOTIONAL SYMPTOMS
- Not marked

WORSE FROM
- Cool bathing or air

BETTER FROM
- Rubbing

VERATRUM ALBUM
(White hellebore)

COMMON AILMENTS
- Diarrhea

- Vomiting

- Collapse

- Painful menstruation

CHARACTERISTIC SYMPTOMS

- Very restless

- Very chilly

- Profuse cold sweat

- Craves juicy, cold drinks and foods

- Cold hands and feet

MENTAL AND EMOTIONAL SYMPTOMS

- Critical and rude

- Jealous

- Haughty, overestimation of own importance

- Lying

- Overstimulated

- Mania and repetitive, compulsive behaviors

WORSE FROM

- Exertion

- Cold drinks (but craves them)

BETTER FROM

- Hot drinks

- Moving

- Warm foods

LIST OF REMEDIES

Aconite (monkshood)
Aesculus (horse chestnut)
Aethusa (fool's parsley)
Allium cepa (red onion)
Aloe (socotrine aloes)
Alumina (aluminum)
Ambrosia (ragweed)
Anacardium (marking nut)
Antimonium crudum (black sulphide of antimony)
Antimonium tartaricum (tartar emetic)
Apis mellifica (crushed honeybee)
Argentum nitricum (silver nitrate)
Arnica montana (mountain daisy or leopard's bane)
Arsenicum album (white arsenic)
Arundo (reed)
Belladonna (deadly nightshade)
Bellis perennis (daisy)
Borax (sodium borate)
Bryonia alba (wild hops)
Calcarea carbonica (Calcium carbonate)
Calcarea phosphorica (Calcium phosphate)
Calendula (marigold)
Cantharis (Spanish fly)
Carbo vegetabilis (vegetable charcoal)
Carbolic acid (phenol)
Causticum (potassium hydrate)
Chamomilla (chamomile)

Chelidonium majus (greater celandine)

China (cinchona or Peruvian bark)

Cimicifuga racemosa (black snakeroot)

Cina (wormseed)

Cocculus (Indian cockle)

Coffea cruda (coffee)

Collinsonia (stoneroot)

Colocynthis (bitter cucumber)

Croton tiglium (croton seed oil)

Cuprum metallicum (copper)

Dioscorea villosa (wild yam)

Drosera (sundew)

Dulcamara (bittersweet)

Equisetum (horsetail)

Eupatorium perfoliatum (boneset)

Euphrasia (eyebright)

Ferrum phosphoricum (iron phosphate)

Gelsemium (yellow jasmine)

Glonoine (nitroglycerine)

Graphites (black lead)

Guaiacum (guaiacum officinale)

Hamamelis (witch hazel)

Hepar sulphuris calcareum (calcium sulphide)

Hydrastis canadensis (goldenseal)

Hypericum (St. John's wort)

Ignatia amara (St. Ignatius bean)

Ipecacuanha (ipecac root)

Iris versicolor (blue flag)

Kali bichromicum (potassium bichromate)

Kali carbonicum (potassium carbonate)

Kali muriaticum (potassium chloride)

Kali phosphoricum (potassium phosphate)

Kreosote (distillation of beechwood tar)

Lachesis (venom of the bushmaster snake)

Ledum palustre (marsh tea or wild rosemary)

Lycopodium (club moss)

Magnesia phosphorica (magnesium phosphate)

Mercurius iodatus flavus (protoiodide of mercury)

Mercurius iodatus ruber (biniodide of mercury)

Mercurius vivus (quicksilver)

Natrum carbonicum (sodium carbonate)

Natrum muriaticum (sodium chloride or common salt)

Natrum sulphuricum (sodium sulphate)

Nitric acid (nitric acid)

Nux vomica (poison nut)

Oscillococcinum (anas barbariae or duck liver and heart)

Petroleum (crude rock oil)

Phosphoric acid (phosphoric acid)

Phosphorus (phosphorus)

Phytolacca (pokeroot)

Podophyllum (mayapple)

Pulsatilla (windflower)

Ratanhia (ratanhia peruviana)

Rhus toxicodendron (poison ivy)

Rumex crispus (yellow dock)

Ruta graveolens (rue)

Sabadilla (cevadilla seed)

Sanguinaria (bloodroot)

Sarsaparilla (smilax)

Sepia (cuttlefish ink)

Silica (pure flint or silicea)

Spigelia (pinkroot)

Spongia tosta (roasted sponge)

Staphysagria (stavesacre)

Stramonium (Thorn apple or jimsonweed)

Strontium carbonicum (strontium carbonate)

Sulphur (sulphur)

Symphytum (comfrey)

Tabacum (tobacco)

Tarentula hispanica (Spanish spider)

Teucrium (cat thyme)
Thuja (arborvitae)
Urtica urens (stinging nettle)
Veratrum album (white hellebore)
Wyethia (poison weed)

GLOSSARY

Acute illness—A self-limiting and short-lived sickness characterized by clear onset and conclusion.

Aggravation—A temporary worsening of existing symptoms that may occur after taking a homeopathic remedy, seen more commonly in treating chronic illness than in first aid or acute situations.

Allopathic medicine—The term used by Samuel Hahnemann to describe conventional medicine: "other suffering." It means that the treatment applied is *opposite* to the condition (antibiotics, antidepressants, antifungal) as distinguished from homeopathy's treating "likes with likes."

Antidote—An influence or factor that disrupts the effectiveness of a homeopathic remedy, slowing, halting, or even reversing it. An antidote can be a substance (e.g., camphor), an emotional shock (e.g., an accident), or an invasive procedure (e.g., oral surgery).

Chronic illness—An illness that is not self-limiting, that has become part of a person's constitution and tends to worsen over time.

Classical homeopathy—A method of homeopathy in which only one remedy is given at a time, its selection based on the patient's total symptom picture, and is given in accordance with the law of similars.

Constitutional treatment—Homeopathic treatment of the whole person in terms of overall health, as opposed to treating acute illness. Constitutional treatment is based upon a carefully taken case history, with the aim of raising the overall level of health, the preventing of illness, or curing a chronic illness.

Cure—A deep and full restoration of health and well-being.

Disease—The result of a weakness or imbalance in the body's defenses that produces limitations to freedom and well-being on physical, emotional, and mental levels.

Healing crisis—A brief intensification of symptoms during the initial phase of the healing process, as the illness is cleared from the body.

Law of cure—Hering's law, which states that during cure the symptoms move from the most important to the least important organs (from the inside to the outside of the body); from above to below (the top of the body to the extremities); and in the reverse order of their appearance.

Materia medica—A reference source containing descriptions of homeopathic remedies, listing symptoms and indications for their use.

Minimum dose—The smallest amount of a homeopathic remedy necessary for healing.

Modality—An influence or factor that makes a particular symptom better or worse.

Mother tincture—A plant extract prepared in an alcohol-based solution from which a potentized homeopathic remedy may be made.

Potency—The strength of a remedy; an indication of the number of times a remedy has been diluted and succussed.

Potentization—The process of preparing homeopathic remedies through progressive dilution and succussion.

Proving—The process by which homeopathic remedies are tested on healthy subjects before they are introduced for therapeutic use.

Remedy—A homeopathic medicine made from a substance that is potentized and then given in accordance with the law of similars.

Remedy picture—The collection of symptoms (mental, emotional, and physical) illustrating the curative powers of a remedy.

Succussion—The vigorous shaking of the remedy solution following each dilution in the process of preparing a homeopathic remedy.

Suppression—When a disturbance or disease is driven deeper into the body, often by an allopathic drug; when symptoms are made to recede or disappear without the vital force being strengthened.

Susceptibility—The predisposition toward a certain type of illness. An inborn or acquired vulnerability.

Symptom picture—The full range of symptoms experienced by a person during illness that is matched to a remedy picture so that the correct homeopathic remedy may be chosen.

Totality of symptoms—A comprehensive picture of a person's illness, representing physical, emotional, and mental characteristics.

Vital force—Samuel Hahnemann's term for the life force or invisible energy that animates all living things. The homeopathic remedy stimulates this force so that the body may heal itself.

SUGGESTED READINGS

GENERAL HOMEOPATHY

Dooley, Timothy. *Homeopathy: Beyond Flat Earth Medicine*.

Gray, Bill. *Homeopathy: Science or Myth?*

Lockie, Andrew, and Nicola Geddes. *The Complete Guide to Homeopathy*.

Reichenberg-Ullman, Judyth, and Robert Ullman. *The Patient's Guide to Homeopathic Medicine*.

Ullman, Dana. *The Consumer's Guide to Homeopathy*.

———. *Discovering Homeopathy: Medicine for the 21st Century*.

Vithoulkas, George. *Homeopathy: Medicine of the New Millennium*.

CHILDREN'S HEALTH

Castro, Miranda. *Homeopathy for Pregnancy, Birth, and Your Baby's First Year*.

Glöcker, Michaela, and Wolfgang Goebel. *A Guide to Child Health*.

Lockie, Andrew. *The Family Guide to Homeopathy*.

Pinto, Gabrielle, and Murray Feldman. *Homeopathy for Children*.

Reichenberg-Ullman, Judyth, and Robert Ullman. *Rage Free Kids*.

———. *Ritalin Free Kids: Homeopathic Treatment of ADD and Other Behavioral and Learning Problems*.

Schmidt, Michael A. *Beyond Antibiotics: 50 (or So) Ways to Boost Immunity and Avoid Antibiotics*.

Uhl, Arlene. *Medicine Moms: Reclaiming Our Children's Health Through Homeopathy*.

Ullman, Dana. *Homeopathic Medicine for Children and Infants*.

WOMEN'S HEALTH

Castro, Miranda. *Homeopathy for Pregnancy, Birth, and Your Baby's First Year.*

Idarius, Betty. *The Homeopathic Childbirth Manual.*

Moskowitz, Richard. *Homeopathic Medicine for Pregnancy and Childbirth.*

Northrup, Christiane. *Women's Bodies, Women's Wisdom.*

Panos, Maisimund, M.D., and Jane Heimlich. *What Homeopathy Can Do for Women.*

Smith, Trevor. *Homeopathic Medicine for Women.*

Speight, Phyllis. *Homeopathic Remedies for Women's Ailments.*

PET HEALTH

Day, Christopher. *Homeopathic Treatment of Small Animals.*

Frazier, Anitra. *The New Natural Cat.*

McCleod, George. *Cats: Homeopathic Remedies.*

———. *Dogs: Homeopathic Remedies.*

Pitcairn, Richard. *Natural Health for Dogs and Cats.*

IMMUNIZATION

Chaitow, Leon. *Vaccination and Immunization: Dangers, Delusions, and Alternatives.*

Coulter, Harris, and Barbara Fisher. *A Shot in the Dark.*

Curtis, Susan. *Handbook of Homeopathic Alternatives to Immunizations.*

Miller, Neil Z. *Vaccines: Are They Really Safe and Effective? A Parent's Guide to Childhood Shots.*

Neustaedter, Randall. *The Vaccine Guide.*

FURTHER STUDY

Bailey, Philip. *Homeopathic Psychology.*

Chappell, Peter. *Emotional Healing with Homeopathy.*

Coulter, Catherine. *Portraits of Homeopathic Medicines*, vols. 1–3.

Coulter, Harris. *Divided Legacy: A History of the Schism in Medical Thought.*

Hahnemann, Samuel. *Organon of the Medical Art,* edited by Wenda Brewster O'Reilly.

Reichenberg-Ullman, Judyth, and Robert Ullman. *Prozac-Free: Homeopathic Medicine for Depression, Anxiety, and Other Mental and Emotional Problems.*

Shepherd, Dorothy. *The Magic of the Minimum Dose.*

Tyler, Margaret. *Homeopathic Drug Pictures.*

Vithoulkas, George. *A New Model for Health and Disease.*

REFERENCE BOOKS

Boericke, W. *Pocket Manual of Homeopathic Materia Medica with Repertory.*

Murphy, Robin. *Homeopathic Medical Repertory,* 2d ed.

Schroyens, Frederik, ed. *Synthesis: Repertorium Homeopathicum Syntheticum.*

Vermeulen, Frans. *Concordant Materia Medica.*

Yasgur, Jay. *Yasgur's Homeopathic Dictionary and Holistic Health Reference,* 4th ed.

BIBLIOGRAPHY

Bailey, Philip M. *Homeopathic Psychology*. Berkeley: North Atlantic Books, 1995.

Castro, Miranda. *The Complete Homeopathy Handbook*. New York: St. Martin's Press, 1991.

Cummings, Stephen, and Dana Ullman. *Everybody's Guide to Homeopathic Medicines*. New York: G. P. Putnam's Sons, 1991.

Glöckler, Michaela, and Wolfgang Goebel. *A Guide to Child Health*. Edinburgh: Floris Books, 1990.

Hahnemann, Samuel. *Organon of the Medical Art*, 6th ed. Edited by Wenda Brewster O'Reilly. Redmond, Wash.: Birdcage Books, 1996.

Kaminski, Patricia. *Flowers That Heal*. Dublin: Newleaf, 1998.

Lockie, Andrew. *The Family Guide to Homeopathy*. New York: Prentice Hall Press, 1989.

Mendelsohn, Robert S. *How to Raise a Healthy Child . . . In Spite of Your Doctor*. Chicago: Contemporary Books, 1984.

Miles, Martin. *Homeopathy and Human Evolution*. London: Winter Press, 1992.

Morrison, Roger. *Desktop Companion*. Nevada City, Calif.: Hahnemann Clinic Publishing, 1998.

———. *Desktop Guide*. Albany, Calif.: Hahnemann Clinic Publishing, 1993.

Murphy, Christine, ed. *Practical Home Care Medicine*. New York: Lantern Books, 2001.

Murphy, Robin. *Homeopathic Medical Repertory*, 2d ed. Pagosa Springs, Colo.: Hahnemann Academy of North America, 1998.

Panos, Maesimund B., and Jane Heimlich. *Homeopathic Medicine at Home*. Los Angeles: J. P. Tarcher, 1980.

Pinto, Gabrielle, and Murray Feldman. *Homeopathy for Children*. Suffolk, United Kingdom: C. W. Daniel Company, 2000.

Smith, Trevor, M.D. *Homeopathic Medicine for Women*. Rochester, Ver.: Healing Arts Press, 1989.

Uhl, Arlene. *Medicine Moms: Reclaiming Our Children's Health Through Homeopathy*. New York: Kensington Publishing, 2001.

Ullman, Dana. *The Consumer's Guide to Homeopathy*. New York: J. P. Tarcher/Putnam, 1995.

———. *Discovering Homeopathy*. Berkeley: North Atlantic Books, 1991.

———. *Homeopathic Medicine for Children and Infants*. New York: J. P. Tarcher/Putnam, 1992.

Ullman, Robert, and Judyth Reichenberg-Ullman. *The Patient's Guide to Homeopathic Medicine*. Edmonds, Wash.: Picnic Point Press, 1995.

Vermeulen, Frans. *Concordant Materia Medica*. Haarlem: Merlijn, 1994.

———. *Synoptic Materia Medica*. Haarlem: Merlijn, 1992.

Vithoulkas, George. *A New Model for Health and Disease*. Mill Valley, Calif.: Health and Habitat, 1991.

———. *The Science of Homeopathy*. New York: Grove Press, 1980.

RESOURCES DIRECTORY

HOMEOPATHIC ORGANIZATIONS

American Institute of Homeopathy (AIH)

WWW.HOMEOPATHYUSA.ORG

801 N. Fairfax Street, Suite 306

Alexandria, VA 22314

Tel.: (888) 445-9988

Periodical: *Journal of the American Institute of Homeopathy*

Council for Homeopathic Certification (CHC)*

WWW.HOMEOPATHICDIRECTORY.COM

P.O. Box 12180

La Crescenta, CA 91224

Tel.: (866) 242-3399

Foundation for Homeopathic Education and Research

2124 Kittredge Street

Berkeley, CA 94704

Tel.: (800) 359-9051

---

* Directory of practitioners available.

Homeopathic Academy of Naturopathic Physicians (HANP)*
WWW.HEALTHY.NET/HANP/
E-mail: info@HANP.org
HANP Database
12132 S.E. Foster Place
Portland, OR 97266
Tel.: (503) 761-3298
Fax: (503) 762-1929
Periodical: *Simillimum*

Homeopathic Nurses' Association
WWW.HOMEOPATHICNURSES.ORG
E-mail: bello@kitcarson.net
HC 81, Box 6023
Questa, NM 87556
Tel.: (800) 530-8800

Homeopaths Without Borders
E-mail: nkeely@igc.org
P.O. Box 570
Bolinas, CA 94924
Tel.: (415) 868-2950

National Center for Homeopathy*
WWW.HOMEOPATHIC.ORG
801 N. Fairfax Street, Suite 306
Alexandria, VA 22314
Tel.: (703) 548-7790
Periodical: *Homeopathy Today*

---

* Directory of practitioners available.

North American Society of Homeopaths (NASH)*
WWW.HOMEOPATHY.ORG
1122 East Pike Street, #1122
Seattle, WA 98122
Tel.: (206) 720-7000
Fax: (206) 329-5684
Periodical: *The American Homeopath*

HOMEOPATHIC PHARMACIES AND SUPPLIERS

Arrowroot Standard Direct
WWW.ARROWROOT.COM
83 E. Lancaster Avenue
Paoli, PA 19301
Tel.: (800) 234-8879

Boericke and Tafel, Inc.
2381 Circadian Way
Santa Rosa, CA 95407
Tel.: (800) 876-9505

Boiron USA
98-C W. Cochran Street
Simi Valley, CA 93065
Tel.: (800) BLU-TUBE

Dolisos America, Inc.
3014 Rigel Avenue
Las Vegas, NV 89102
Tel.: (800) 365-4767

---

* Directory of practitioners available.

Hahnemann Laboratories, Inc.
WWW.HAHNEMANNLABS.COM
1940 Fourth Street
San Rafael, CA 94901
Tel.: (888) 427-6422

Heel Inc.
WWW.HEELBHI.COM
11600 Cochiti S.E.
Albuquerque, NM 87123
Tel.: (800) 621-7644

Helios Pharmacy U.K.
WWW.HELIOS.CO.UK
97 Camden Road
Tunbridge Wells, Kent TN1 2QR, U.K.
Tel.: (01892) 536393

Homeopathic Educational Services
WWW.HOMEOPATHIC.COM/INDEX.HTML
2124 Kittredge Street
Berkeley, CA 94704
Tel.: (510) 649-0294

Luytes Pharmacal Co.
4200 Laclede Street
St. Louis, MO 63108
Tel.: (800) Homeopathy

Natural Health Supply
WWW.A2ZHOMEOPATHY.COM
6410 Avenida Christina
Santa Fe, NM 87505
Tel.: (888) 689-1608

Standard Homeopathic Co.
210 W. 131st Street
Los Angeles, CA 90061
Tel.: (800) 624-9659

Washington Homeopathic Products, Inc.
WWW.HOMEOPATHYWORKS.COM
4914 Delray Avenue
Bethesda, MD 20814
Tel.: (301) 656-1695

Weleda, Inc.
WWW.WELEDA.COM
175 North Route 9W
Congers, NY 10920
Tel.: (800) 241-1030

HOMEOPATHIC TRAINING PROGRAMS
Bastyr University
E-mail: admiss@bastyr.edu
14500 Juanita Drive, N.E.
Kenmore, WA 98028-4966
Tel.: (425) 823-1300

Hahnemann College of Homeopathy
WWW.HAHNEMANNCOLLEGE.COM
80 Nicholl Avenue
Point Richmond, CA 94801
Tel.: (510) 232-2079
Fax: (510) 412-9044

Institute of Classical Homeopathy
1336-D Oak Avenue
St. Helena, CA 94574
Tel.: (415) 248-1632

National College of Naturopathic Medicine
WWW.NCNM.EDU
11231 S.E. Market Street
Portland, OR 97216
Tel.: (503) 255-4860

New England School of Homeopathy
WWW.NESH.COM
356 Middle Street
Amherst, MA 01002
Tel.: (413) 256-5949

Northwest Academy of Homeopathy
E-mail: remedy@mnn.net
10700 Old Country Road #15, Suite 300
Plymouth, MN 55441
Tel.: (612) 794-6445

Pacific Academy of Homeopathy
E-mail: pahm@slip.net
1199 Sanchez Street
San Francisco, CA 94114
Tel.: (415) 458-8238
Fax: (415) 695-8220

The School of Homeopathy, Devon, England
WWW.HOMEOPATHYSCHOOL.COM
82 East Pearl Street
New Haven, CT 06513
Tel.: (203) 624-8783

The School of Homeopathy, New York
WWW.HOMEOPATHYSCHOOL.COM
964 Third Avenue, 8th Floor
New York, NY 10155-0003
Tel.: (212) 570-2576

Southwest College of Naturopathic Medicine
WWW.SCNM.EDU
2140 East Broadway Road
Tempe, AZ 85282
Tel.: (602) 858-9100
Fax: (602) 858-9116

Teleosis School of Homeopathy
WWW.TELEOSIS.COM
333 W. 56th Street, #1C
New York, NY 10019
Tel.: (212) 977-8118

Vancouver Homeopathic Academy
WWW.HOMEOPATHYVANCOUVER.COM
P.O. Box 34095 Station D
Vancouver, BC, Canada
Tel.: (604) 708-9387
Fax: (604) 708-1547

HOMEOPATHY RESOURCES ON THE INTERNET
Baltimore Homeopathy Study Group
WWW.BALTIMORE-HOMEOPATHY.ORG
An informative site featuring a remedy quiz.

Similia Similibus
WWW.CURANTUR.DE
An educational site containing classic texts and articles.

HomeopathyFAQ

WWW.HOMEOPATHYFAQ.COM

Articles for those interested in serious study.

Homeopathy for Women's and Children's Health

WWW.SABER.NET/~BIDARIUS/HOMEO

A site created by homeopaths Miranda Castro and Betty Idarius.

Homeopathy Home Page

WWW.HOMEOPATHYHOME.COM

One of the most complete homeopathic references on the Web. A great starting point for finding factual and accurate information about homeopathy.

Homeopathic Online Education

WWW.SIMILLIMUM.COM

An educational site created by homeopath David Little.

Homeopathic Website

WWW.SIMILLIBUS.COM

Resources, articles, and links, including a directory of practitioners; created by homeopath Will Taylor, M.D.

Homeopathy On-Line Magazine

WWW.LYGHTFORCE.COM

National Center for Homeopathy

WWW.HOMEOPATHIC.ORG

ON-LINE MAILING LISTS AND DISCUSSION GROUPS

These lists are generally educational and do not encourage questions about specific ailments from the public. They are very useful for students and others who wish to learn more about homeopathy and participate interactively.

Holistic Discussion Group

WWW.HOMEOPATHYHOME.COM/WEB/DESCRIPTIONS/HOLIS.
SHTML

Homeopathy Mailing List

WWW.HOMEOPATHYHOME.COM/WEB/DESCRIPTIONS/HOMLIST.
SHTML

HOMEOPATHIC BOOK SOURCES

Homeopathic Educational Services

WWW.HOMEOPATHIC.COM

2124 Kittredge Street
Berkeley, CA 94704
Tel.: (800) 359-9051

Minimum Price Books

WWW.MINIMUM.COM

250 H Street
P.O. Box 2187
Blaine, WA 98231
Tel.: (800) 663-8272

North Atlantic Books

WWW.NORTHATLANTICBOOKS.COM

1456 Fourth Street
Berkeley, CA 94710
Tel.: (800) 337-BOOK

HOMEOPATHIC SOFTWARE PROGRAMS

CARA
C.H.I.R.O.N. Software
E-mail: chiron@chiron-h.com
1044 Water Street
Port Townsend, WA 98368
Tel.: (360) 385-1926

MacRepertory and Reference Works
Kent Homeopathic Associates
WWW.KENTHOMEOPATHIC.COM
710 Mission Avenue
San Rafael, CA 94901
Tel.: (877) 937-5368

RADAR
Whole Health Now
WWW.WHOLEHEALTHNOW.COM
1102 Pleasant Street, PMB816
Worcester, MA 01602
Tel.: (508) 756-2987

INDEX

Note: Bold page numbers refer to major discussions of topic.

Ben-Gay, 37
bioflavonoids, 98, 103
bites and stings
  animal, 47, 55, **85–87**
  dosage and potency for, 32–33,
    55
  and hives, 167, 168
  human, 85, 86, 87
  insect, 32–33, 46, 47, 48, 55,
    81–85, 167, 168
  remedies for, 46, 47, 48, 81–85,
    232, 255, 256
bladder conditions, 32–33, 59,
  185–88. *See also* bed-wetting
bleeding, **59–61**
  and bites and stings, 83, 86
  and circumcision, 203–4
  and dosage and potency for first
    aid, 55, 56
  and eye injuries, 71
  and fainting, 72
  and fractured bones, 76
  and head injuries, 77, 78
  and hemorrhoids, 149, 150
  and puncture wounds, 86
  remedies for, 55, 56, 57, 60
  and teething, 222
  and warts, 173, 174
  See also blood; nosebleeds
blisters, **61,** 64, 66, 101, 102, 170,
  171, 172, 201
Blistex, 37
blood
  dark, 83
  loss of, 72
  sight of, 72, 73
  in urine, 186, 187, 188
  vomiting of, 129
  See also bleeding
blows, 58, 62, 71, 77, 219

boils, **165,** 210–11, 249, 255
bones
  broken, 33–34, 57
  bruised, 91
  crushed, 75
  and eye injuries, 71
  fractured, **74–76**
  weak or brittle, 74
boneset. See *Eupatorium perfoliatum*
Borax, 102, 160, 191, 222
bowel or bladder control, 59. *See
  also* constipation; diarrhea
breast-feeding, 205, 206
bronchitis, **104–5, 111–15,** 129,
  202
bruises, **62**
  and bites and stings, 83
  and bleeding, 60
  causes of, 62
  and dosage and potency for first
    aid, 55, 56
  and eye/vision problems, 70
  and fractured bones, 74, 76
  and head injuries, 76, 77
  remedies for, 46, 48, 55, 56, 57,
    62, 90, 233
  and sprains, strains, and soreness,
    90, 91
Bryonia alba, **237–38**
  and abdominal pain, 117
  and appendicitis, 100
  and back injuries and backaches,
    58, 237
  and colds, coughs, and
    bronchitis, 109, 112
  and constipation, 120
  and digestive problems, 126, 237
  and fever, 137
  and fractured bones, 74
  and headaches, 142–43, 237

cramps (*cont'd*)
  and heat exhaustion/sunstroke,
    80
  and indigestion, 127
  menstrual, 185, **188–91**
  muscle, 79
  and nausea and vomiting, 129
  remedies for, 48
cranberry juice, 187
creams/ointments, 45. *See also type
  of cream/ointment*
Croton tiglium, 170
croup, 108, 111, **211–13**
Cullen, William, 5–6
Cuprum metallicum, 80
cures, **15–18**
cuts and scrapes, 46, 47, 48, 56,
  67–68, 71, 76
cuttlefish ink. See *Sepia*
cystitis (bladder infection),
  185–88, 232, 268

dental work, 38, 175, 182–84
depression, 77, **134–35,** 192, 268
diagnosis. *See* case taking; reviewing
  findings
diaper rash, 46, **214**
diarrhea, **122–25**
  and abdominal pain, 116, 117,
    118
  and colic, 204, 205
  as digestive problem, 115
  dosage and potency for, 33
  and food poisoning, 141
  and heat exhaustion/sunstroke,
    80
  and hives, 168
  and indigestion, 127
  and influenza, 151, 153

  and mental and emotional
    condition, 132
  and nausea and vomiting, 128,
    129
  remedies for, 33, 122–25, 234,
    241, 258, 265, 272, 274
  and teething, 221
  travelers', 123
diet
  and creating a healing
    atmosphere, **49**
  See also specific condition
digestive problems, **115–30**
  and fever, 135, 138
  and hives, 168
  and influenza, 153
  and insomnia, 156
  remedies for, 48, 234, 237, 257,
    258, 260, 261, 263, 265
  See also specific problem
Dioscorea villosa, 205
dosage
  and administering remedies, 40
  and assessing response to
    remedies, 35
  for first aid, **55–56**
  frequency for administering, 32,
    34, 38, 40
  guidelines for, **32–34**
  minimum, **7,** 32
  selecting, **31–34**
Drosera, 109, 212–13
drowning, **68–69**
drugs
  allergies to, 168, 169
  avoiding, 38
  and colds, 108
  and diarrhea, 124
  and fever, 138

and injuries, 58, 77, 250
as lotion/tincture, 47, 61, 86–87, 167, 209
and mental and emotional symptoms, 250
and seizures, 250
and skin problems, 166
and splinters, 89
and surgery, 175
and tetanus, 87
and tooth pain, 184
and wounds, 85–87, 250
hysteria. *See* mental and emotional conditions

ice packs, 48, 59, 61, 71, 78, 84, 92
Ignatia amara, 44, 73, 134, 143, 149, 155, 178, 189, **251–52**
illness
factors leading to, 14
onset and chronology of, **24**
past, 36
as time of cleansing, 49
uniqueness of individual's, 21–22
and vital force, 13
what is, **14–15**
immune system, 10, 12–13, 15, 17–18, 197–99
impotence, 257
indian cockle. See *Cocculus indica*
indigestion, **126–28**, 147
infections, 4, 47, 85–87, 249. *See also type of infection*
inflammation, 47, 59, 229, 247. *See also type of inflammation*
influenza, **151–53**
and diarrhea, 122, 123
and fever, 137, 138
and headaches, 143
and nausea and vomiting, 128

remedies for, 48, 151–53, 234, 235, 237, 245, 247, 262
and throat complaints, 180
injuries
as condition treated by homeopathy, 4
crushing, 62, 75
and dosage and potency for first aid, 55
and Hering's law, 16, 17
and nosebleeds, 219
past, 17
remedies for, 47, 48, 57, 58, 233, 270
See also type of injury
insomnia, 5, 135, 138, **153–57,** 183, 203, 243, 244
intuition, 25
ipecac root. See *Ipecacuanha*
Ipecacuanha, 44, 60, 113, 123, 129, 144, **252–53**
Ipsab herbal gum treatment, 103, 184
Iris versicolor, 144
iron phosphate. See *Ferrum phosphoricum*
irritability. *See* mental and emotional symptoms; *specific condition*
itching. *See specific condition*

jet lag, **157–58,** 233, 243

Kali bichromicum, 107–8, 110, 144, 159, 165, **253–54**
Kali carbonicum, 113, 114, **254–55**
Kali muriaticum, 223
Kali phosphoricum, 155
kitchen remedies, 42, **48**
Kreosote, 192, 200, 222

muscle problems (*cont'd*)
  and pain, 48, 90, 237
  pulled, 90
  sore, 46, 56
  stiff, 56
  See also sprains; strains

nails, 86, 101, 270
Natrum carbonicum, 80
Natrum muriaticum, 97, 102,
  134–35, 145, **260–61**
Natrum sulphuricum, 77–78
nausea, **128–30**
  and abdominal pain, 118
  and appendicitis, 99
  and back injuries and backaches,
    59, 60
  and chicken pox, 202
  and colds, coughs, and
    bronchitis, 109, 113
  and diarrhea, 123
  and digestive problems, 115,
    127
  and food poisoning, 141
  and headaches, 143, 144, 145
  and heat exhaustion/sunstroke,
    79, 80, 81
  and influenza, 128
  and motion sickness, 160, 161,
    162
  remedies for, 128–30, 252
  and surgery, 175
  and women's ailments, 189, 190
neck problems, 77, 140, 148, 180,
  250, 267
nerves, 58, 62, 77, 87, 123, 175, 250
neti pot, 99, 164
news, bad/shocking, 30, 247, 251,
  260

Nitric acid, 173
nose, 96, 97, 98. *See also* nosebleeds;
  sneezing; *specific condition*
nosebleeds, 59, 60, 110, 113, 114,
  219–20, 263
Noxzema, 37
Nux vomica, **261–63**
  and abdominal pain, 119
  and allergies and hay fever, 97,
    262
  and bladder infections, 186
  and colds, 108, 261
  and colic, 206, 262
  and constipation, 120–21
  and diarrhea, 124
  and digestive problems, 127, 261
  and fainting, 73
  and fever, 138
  and food poisoning, 141
  and hangovers, 262
  and headaches, 145–46
  and hemorrhoids, 149
  and hives, 168
  in home kit, 44
  and influenza, 152–53, 262
  and insomnia, 155
  and mental and emotional
    conditions, 130–31, 262
  and motion sickness, 161
  and nausea and vomiting, 129
  and PMS/menstrual cramps,
    189
  and sore throats, 262

oatmeal baths, 172, 203
observation, and case taking, 22,
  25–27
onions, 48, 126, 217–18. See also
  Allium cepa

ABOUT THE AUTHOR

LAURA JOSEPHSON, C.C.H., R.S.Hom. (NA), has been in homeopathic practice since 1992. She is currently the president of the New York State Homeopathic Association. Her interest in homeopathy grew out of her study of herbology and hermetic science. She has studied at the New York School of Homeopathy, the Atlantic Academy of Classical Homeopathy, the New England School of Homeopathy, and with various leaders in the field from around the world. A native of Northern California, she maintains a private practice in Rockland County, New York, where she lives with her husband, four daughters, and a menagerie of dogs, cats, and birds.